EASY FITNESS FOR QUITTERS

Katie Mackenzie

 MAJOLIER PRESS

ISBN: 978-1-7392324-0-5 (paperback)

ISBN: 978-1-7392324-1-2 (ebook)

This publication is designed to provide accurate information in regard to the subject matter covered. The information in this book was correct at the time of publication, but the author does not assume any liability for loss or damage caused by errors or omissions.

The advice and strategies contained herein may not be suitable for your situation. This book does not replace the advice of a medical professional. Consult your physician before making any changes to your regular health plan.

Book Cover and illustrations by Katie Mackenzie, except cover elements, including the shoes, which are from canva.com.

Printed in the United Kingdom

First edition 2022

Visit the author's website at www.easyfitnessforquitters.com.

To everyone who would rather not.

And of course to the wonderful R, Z and S. You're the best.

BEFORE WE START

All the advice in this book is very general, and not designed to constitute a training plan. Nothing in this book is medical advice and is not to be taken as such.

You know your own body, and the aim is to help you work with what you've got, what you enjoy and what you feel comfortable doing.

If you have any concerns about your mental or physical health or ability to perform any kind of movement, please speak to a health professional.

CONTENTS

Introduction: On being a quitter

I am not a fitness guru or a gym bunny. As soon as a personal trainer tells me that a class is going to be 'fun', I'm on the lookout for the nearest exit. I am not much of a runner, but I will happily run away from the gym. I have lost count of all the different exercise classes and new fitness regimes I've tried over the years. So why is a quitter like me writing a book about fitness, and why should you read it?

Well, I'm not a quitter any more. I have found forms of exercise I genuinely enjoy and can see myself carrying on for as long as I'm physically able. I also accept that I am doing enough, even if it might not look like what we have been led to believe 'keeping fit' should look like. You can reach this point too, I promise.

Almost everyone I've ever seen encouraging people to exercise is someone who is already sold on the whole fitness scene. The books I've read about health and fitness are by people who study exercise or movement because they love it, or casually mention that they used to do a sport competitively. These people may know the science behind why we should exercise, and they know what the benefits are, but they don't really speak to those of us who have never seen ourselves as sporty. This is a fitness book for people who don't want anything to do with fitness.

Whether we are sporty or not, we all want to live a full and healthy life for as long as possible, and being physically active is one of the best ways to improve our chances of doing so. You cannot have missed being told to do more exercise, so why is it we lack motivation to do something that is patently so good for us?

Humans are cunning and lazy

Going to a spin class is against human nature. It's not actually natural to want to exercise. After all, it's not uncommon for humans to prefer to do the things that are bad for us, is it?

When it comes to exercise, the reason we don't want to do it is because of our history as a species. While our modern lives are probably as stressful as they have ever been, in purely movement terms, we are incredibly physically comfortable. Compared to our ancestors, our houses are dry and easy to heat. We have hot showers and squishy sofas; our clothes and shoes protect us from the elements and the environment. We can order almost anything we want and have it delivered to our door with little more than lifting a single finger and gently stroking it a couple of times on a smooth phone screen.

Of course, not everybody has it this easy. Not everyone has a warm comfortable home that they can afford to heat, but the level of comfort and inactivity we expect as the norm would be completely alien to early humans. I'm sure a cave woman would be absolutely delighted by a bubble bath and a piping hot curry delivered to her door. Let's be honest, as a species, humans are too clever. We devise absolutely marvellous inventions to allow us to do as little physical work as possible.

It is completely rational to conserve energy. All species do it: have you *seen* cats? They don't move if they don't have to. Humans are no different. When you consider that if you live in a place or time where food is relatively scarce because you have to catch it or forage for it yourself, you would be very unwise to go skipping about burning calories unnecessarily. Why use precious energy stores on a spin class? It's much more sensible to do the bare minimum so that you have the reserves to get more food when you need it, and so that you can reproduce and carry on the species. Don't be hard on yourself for not getting up at 5:30am to go for a bracing jog in the gloom and drizzle. Your ancestors wouldn't have fancied it either.

However, this leaves us in a bit of a predicament: exercise and movement are really, really good for us. Until recently, we have needed to move our bodies and use our muscles to fulfil our most basic requirements. There are enormous benefits to being fit and reasonably active, but we have designed our lifestyles to allow us to move as little as possible. Why should we fight against our nature to get fit? And how can we do it in such a way that it doesn't feel like a fight?

Feeling better about yourself

Exercise and diet often go hand in hand for people looking to achieve a healthier lifestyle, especially if that involves losing weight. Many of us only try to exercise to get slimmer and then give up when it doesn't work. However, fitness isn't like a diet and for me, the two things are quite separate. This is not a 'how to lose weight' book, it is a 'how to move more' book. With moving more, you're not denying yourself anything, and throughout this book we will explore how to make exercise not feel like exercise. It could even be pleasant! Weight loss might be a side effect, but I'm not making any promises and, as you will see, the benefits of getting more movement into your life are considerably broader than dropping a few pounds. Plus, if you like yourself more, perhaps it's not so important what the numbers on the scales say.

I will help you stop feeling guilty about not doing enough exercise, and to stop feeling like it is something that you are bad at. You will feel motivated to move more and don't worry, it is surprisingly easy to improve your fitness, with minimal time and effort. Being 'fit enough' is achievable.

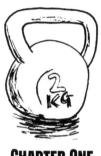

CHAPTER ONE

WHAT IS THE POINT OF GETTING MORE EXERCISE?

What is 'fit'?

First things first, what do we mean when we talk about fitness? Is there a certain level of strength, endurance or speed we need to achieve to be considered fit?

There are various tests to measure how well your heart and lungs cope with being made to work harder. You can count how many push-ups you can do, or your resting heart rate. You could see how fast you can run or walk a mile. But the easiest test of all is probably the question: do you feel fit?

If you are reading this because you don't feel fit and you want to get fitter, it doesn't particularly matter how you score on any of the tests. You know if you're unfit. You know how out of breath you get climbing stairs or how hard you find it to carry heavy bags.

My Great Uncle Jim lived in the Lake District. He was a mountain guide, climbing instructor, and a founder of the first organised Lake District mountain rescue team. Every morning before breakfast, he would walk up the Coniston Old Man and back. Apparently, it took him an hour and a half. That was before the day's work of walking up and down hills as a guide. Jim's nephew, my Uncle Jeremy, who in his day was the fittest person I've ever known, said when he was a young man he asked Jim if he could go with him one morning. "Are you fit?" Jim asked. Jeremy managed it in 1 hour 45 minutes, and he had to run back down. He excused his 'poor' performance by saying that on the way up he helped another man who was struggling. I've not walked the Coniston Old Man myself, but Google tells me to allow between 4 and a half and 6 hours to do it. It's just over 8 and a half miles. If legend is to be believed, Great Uncle Jim was charging up and down the Old Man at a pace of around a ten and a half minute mile. That's the speed I jog on a flat pavement (and I certainly can't maintain that pace for 8 miles). So if you were to ask your great niece the same question, Great Uncle Jim, my answer would be: "by your standards, no, I am not 'fit'."

But I don't need to be *that* fit. I'm not a professional mountain guide in the Lake District whose livelihood depends on being able to walk up and down mountains all day. There's a very wide spectrum between completely sedentary and Great Uncle Jim. You and I are probably some way off being as fit as someone who runs about for their job, but don't be demoralised. We don't need to be.

What is the difference between movement and exercise?

'Exercise' is not a word that fills us quitters with enthusiasm. To make sure that we're all talking about the same thing, 'exercise' is training particular muscles or the cardiovascular system by performing specific movements, often repetitively. It's an activity you do with the express purpose of making your body strong and healthy. If you have an injury or weakness in a certain area, you can do exercises to improve it.

One problem with being a grownup is nobody is forcing you to do this stuff any more. If you're anything like me, you have memories of standing, freezing, on the school hockey pitch, hoping to God that no one wallops the ball towards your numb-with-cold knuckles. Or cross country 'running' where you puffed and panted at the back, wondering if you have developed asthma in the last ten minutes, while some fresh-looking girl laps you with barely a glossy hair out of place.

In whatever free time we have, however little that might be, we have so many ways to entertain ourselves while slumped on a sofa, and so few PE teachers shouting at us to "DON'T STOP! KEEP RUNNING!" Maybe that's the answer: all we need is to hire someone to stand beside our sofas and yell at us if we sit on them.

Movement, on the other hand, is not done for physical improvement. You move to do other things, like gardening. Raking up an enormous pile of leaves, lifting them into the wheelie bin and moving the heavy bin around is all movement, and may replicate a lot of things you might do for exercise in the gym. You'll work the same muscles, but you're not doing it for exercise, you're doing it because the leaves need raking. You could go out into your garden right now and dig a big hole to plant a tree in. That would exercise your muscles (and probably hurt your back) but it's not what we would traditionally think of as 'exercise'. If someone asks you what you do to keep fit, they might give you a funny look if you said you like to dig holes. Try telling that to strangers at parties.

We're going to look at both movement and exercise in the next few chapters, but let's start by looking at exercise. Do you know why exactly exercise is so good for you? We are used to being told that exercise is good for our hearts, but there is actually a bit more to it than that, and I think it's helpful to look at the many ways it benefits our bodies.

Why exercise at all?

Many of us in the Western world are becoming increasingly sedentary, as we spend more time sitting and less time being physically active than previous generations. But is that really a problem? Our life expectancy is as long as it's ever been and we can get by just fine without exercising, can't we? Unfortunately, countries like the UK are seeing big increases in so-called 'lifestyle' diseases. These are diseases that cause illness and early death that are to a large extent preventable by having a healthy lifestyle.

An unhealthy lifestyle can "result in the development of chronic diseases, specifically heart disease, stroke, diabetes, obesity, metabolic syndrome, chronic obstructive pulmonary disease, and some types of cancer."[1] The top three risk factors are smoking, unhealthy diet and... you've guessed it: being sedentary.

Perhaps lifestyle diseases only appear to be a problem because not nearly as many of us die in infancy or in childbirth, or from infections and diseases that were deadly before the invention of antibiotics and vaccines. That's partly true, but there is no reason to think that getting type-2 diabetes is something that should be considered normal, yet the NHS describes it as a "common condition".[2] Type-2 diabetes can cause serious health issues that permanently damage your body, but changes to diet and exercise levels greatly reduce the risk of developing it.

We have treatments for many diseases like heart disease or cancer, but the treatments themselves are not without undesirable side effects. You might survive a stroke. You might live just as long as you would have done if you hadn't developed the type-2 diabetes. But consider your quality of life. If you're going to live for a long time, you want to aim to enjoy your later years, not to spend those years limited by and suffering from diseases that might have been avoided.

Of course, it's not guaranteed that if you live a healthy lifestyle you're going to live a long, pain-free life. No one can make that promise. But you can improve your odds. The more you exercise, the longer your life expectancy. The older you get, the stronger the relationship between exercise and staying alive becomes. If you're getting on a bit, this is no time to start slacking as it's more important than ever to keep active. In *Exercised*, Professor Daniel Lieberman states that according to a study of over seventeen thousand university alumni carried out over twenty years,

> "Middle-aged alumni who exercised more than two thousand calories per week had a 21 percent lower risk of dying than their sedentary classmates, and those who were over seventy and exercised the same amount had half the risk of dying in a given year as their inactive classmates. Yes, half."[3]

Study after study has shown that moderate exercise is good for you, and even a small amount of exercise reduces your risk of dying, compared with doing no exercise at all. If you start exercising now, and keep it up, you've got a much better chance of being able to do the things you enjoy, be around the people you love, and visit the places you want to go for many years to come.

Moderate exercise also helps reduce levels of inflammation in your body. Western diets, stress, disease, too much body fat (especially around the organs), can all cause low levels of inflammation to persist in your body, maybe for years. Inflammation is a natural and beneficial process whereby we fight off infection and heal wounds. It is your internal defence system, which normally provides a short-lived and vigorous response to a wound or a cold virus. There's redness, swelling and, if it's a cold, snot. But many people have low levels of chronic inflammation hanging around in their systems, and links have been found between chronic inflammation and depression[4] and a host of other problems:

> "In the last decade, chronic inflammation has been strongly implicated as a major cause of dozens of noninfectious diseases associated with aging, including heart disease, type 2 diabetes, and Alzheimer's. The more we look, the more we find the fingerprints of chronic inflammation on

yet more diseases including colon cancer, lupus, multiple sclerosis, and just about every medical condition with the suffix '-itis' including arthritis."[5]

When you do moderate exercise, your body can reduce levels of inflammation in your system at the same time as it repairs the tired muscles. Muscles become inflamed when exercised and so there is a corresponding anti-inflammatory response. The healing process is indiscriminate, it doesn't just work on the muscles in isolation. Please note, there are other ways of lowering inflammation too, such as through diet or medication. Talk to your doctor about it if you are concerned, because there may be an underlying cause of the inflammation that needs treating, and exercise might not be an appropriate treatment. I think of it as a useful protective measure.

Another anecdote from a relative: my Granny Peggy was active all her life. She loved gardening and playing golf. She liked a walk and was always keen to be outdoors and active. I remember her stomp of a walk fondly. She was still working part time and playing golf in her nineties, with few health complaints, until one day she was getting out of a friend's car at the golf club, too slowly, considering what happened next. Her friend didn't realise she was still there and drove off, straight onto her ankle. When asked if she was OK, my never-before-known-to-swear Granny's response was, "Yes, when you get this fucking car off my ankle."

The period of immobility that followed caused a precipitous decline. I'm sure you have come across similar stories of elderly people who were fine until they had a fall, then it all went wrong. Not long after the broken ankle, Peggy's short-term memory started to go. She couldn't remember what she had just said or done. Had she not been run over, we're convinced she would have made it to the age of one hundred. As it happened, she only made it to 99 and a third.

Periods of inactivity, such as bed rest, are called 'deconditioning' and can lead to many problems if steps aren't taken to regain muscle strength. Many studies have concluded that,

> "...long periods of immobility are detrimental to the health of all body systems, and also that inactivity is an important factor in the development of chronic-degenerative diseases..."[6]

It's a problem for astronauts, the elderly, and the sedentary. If you have to go into hospital they try to get you up and about as quickly as possible, not just because they want the bed back for the next patient, but also because it's well known that you will get better faster if you move. How on earth Uncle Joe in *Charlie and the Chocolate Factory* jumped up to take a tour of the chocolate factory after all those years of lying in bed, I do not know. I reckon he must have been doing some circuits around the block at night.

Moving for your mood

Exercise is just one tool in the mental health toolkit and it may not be appropriate for everyone and every condition. But to boost your mood, it well known that exercise is at least as good as many anti-depressant drugs at treating mild to moderate depression.

In the UK, GPs can and do prescribe exercise to help with depression and low mood, as well as other conditions. The National Institute for Health and Care Excellence (NICE) recommends that people with mild to moderate depression take part in about three sessions of exercise a week. The reason exercise is thought to be helpful is because exercising spurs the release of proteins called neurotrophic or growth factors. These cause nerve cells to grow and make new connections. The new connections in the hippocampus (where mood is regulated) make your brain better able to regulate your mood.[7]

What sort of exercise should I be doing?

All this makes it clear that exercise protects against lifestyle diseases, reduces inflammation, helps you live longer, and boosts your mood. But there are so many different types of exercise, none of which particularly appeal. So if I'm going to do some, where should I start?

We can break exercise as an activity down into two broad areas: endurance and strength. Many forms of keeping fit involve an element of both. For example, you need both endurance and muscle strength to swim for half an hour, or to hike up a steep hill.

You will have heard people talk about 'cardio', or 'aerobic exercise', which is what I mean by 'endurance'. This is sustained movement that gets your heart pumping and you breathe harder. Remember aerobics videos from the 80s? It's that. It is also things like jogging, brisk walking, swimming, or cycling. Cardio is really just moving around faster and for longer than normal, and you don't have to wear a leotard and legwarmers to do it.

· · • ••·•••· · ·

Why do aerobic exercise?
- It strengthens your heart muscles – During exercise, your body sends oxygen to your muscles faster, so the heart muscles strengthen, meaning it can pump more blood with each beat.

- It improves circulation – Aerobic exercise increases the volume of plasma in the blood, allowing the heart to pump blood more easily. Arteries and capillaries expand.

- It raises good cholesterol and lowers bad cholesterol

- It *helps keep resting blood pressure and heart rate low*

- It *promotes the growth of muscle*

- It *burns fat and improves the body's ability to use sugars*

- It *lowers levels of inflammation*

- It *adjusts the levels of hormones*

- It *stimulates bones to grow and repair*

- It *strengthens connective tissues – including tendons, ligaments and cartilage.*

- *Moderate exercise stimulates the immune system, helping to fight off diseases – though you should rest if you're already suffering from an infection.*

- It *increases blood flow to the brain, stimulating brain cell growth, maintenance and function*

- *Being active as you age can slow the onset of dementia*

··•••·•••··

We didn't evolve to be super strong with big, bulging muscles like gorillas, but we need strength and power as well as endurance. If you look at modern hunter-gatherer peoples, they tend more towards wiry and lean, rather than bulky.

Strength is how much force you can produce, and power is how fast you can produce it, so it's not just about how heavy a weight you can lift, but also can you jump over a puddle? Can you repeatedly lift something, like digging that big hole in your garden? We need power for running and jumping and we need strength for lifting and carrying.

With strength, it is absolutely a case of use it or lose it. As we get older (past the age of 40) our muscle fibres decrease in size and number, and our nerves degenerate, meaning that we lose strength. Our bones also deteriorate. For women, oestrogen has a protective effect on your bones, so once you are post-menopause, the lack of oestrogen makes this bone loss extra risky. Once you start losing strength, it can become a steady decline into not being able to get up from a chair, climb the stairs, or carry a bag of shopping. The weaker you become, the less active you feel like being, which just makes the problem worse. If you are weaker and use your body less, you are at greater risk of osteoporosis, and the other diseases mentioned earlier. However, whatever age you are, your muscles will respond to training, and you don't have to accept becoming feeble when old. According to Wikipedia, the world record for a mile run for an 85-year-old man is six minutes, 40 seconds, and for an 85-year-old woman is ten minutes, 55 seconds. That gives me a few decades to work on improving my mile run time.

・・・●・●・●・・

What benefits will I get from being stronger?

- *Stronger bones and joints. Weight-bearing activities put forces onto your bones, joints and muscles, which cause the cells to activate and build back stronger. Lifting heavy weights or running place loads onto the bones and will help you develop a stronger skeleton. Low-impact activities like swimming or cycling don't have the same benefits for your bones. Post-menopausal women especially need to focus on loading their bones to keep them strong.*

- *Building strength and power helps your endurance. Any serious runner or cyclist does weight training and power training (called plyometrics - it's a lot of jumping onto boxes). It gets your muscles to adapt faster so they are better able to use oxygen, which will really help you if you are interested in improving your endurance.*

- *Strength training improves your cardiovascular fitness, just like endurance training does, giving you the associated benefits to your heart, etc.*

- *Muscles help manage blood sugar levels. When*

you use your muscles during weight training, they pull glucose from the bloodstream, keeping blood sugar levels from rising dangerously high. The American Diabetes Association recommends that anyone with insulin resistance or diabetes practises strength training twice a week or more.

- Strength training helps control your weight. A regular strength training regime slows weight gain, decreases waist circumference, and reduces the amount of dangerous fat around the organs.

- It improves your joint flexibility. Amazingly, strength training appears to be better than stretching for improving joint flexibility.

- It decreases your risk of falls and injury. Having stronger muscles will support your joints and skeleton, so even if you have weakness or arthritis in your knees, for example, your muscles will keep you upright and take the pressure off the problem areas. This is why physiotherapists give you muscle strengthening exercises to deal with a dodgy shoulder or wonky hip.

••••••••••

Getting fit is easier than you think

There is a huge list of advantages to be gained from exercising, but it might surprise you to discover that you don't need to do very much exercise to get these benefits.

If you're thinking you've got to be finding an hour a day to do something horribly sweaty and unpleasant, the absolutely brilliant news is that this isn't the case AT ALL:

> "The health benefits of activity follow, in fact, a breathtakingly steep curve at first... In a recent meta-analysis of studies about exercise and mortality conducted by scientists at the University of Cambridge and others, the authors found that in general a person's risk of dying prematurely from any cause plummeted by nearly 20 percent if he or she began to meet the current exercise guidelines of 150 minutes of moderate activity per week, compared with someone who didn't exercise."[8]

The less exercise you currently do, the more you have to gain by even the smallest incremental increase in activity. It doesn't matter how old or unfit you are.

Just do a bit. It may feel hard at first, but your body will adapt to it. Then you can do a bit more.

· · · ● · ● ● · ● · · ·

What is the current advice on exercise?

Different governments have produced broadly similar guidelines on the quantity of exercise we ought to do. The NHS UK says "adults should aim to:

- do strengthening activities that work all the major muscle groups (legs, hips, back, abdomen, chest, shoulders and arms) on at least two days a week

- do at least 150 minutes of moderate intensity activity a week or 75 minutes of vigorous intensity activity a week

- spread exercise evenly over four to five days a week, or every day

- reduce time spent sitting or lying down and break up long periods of not moving with some activity

You can also achieve your weekly activity target with:
- several short sessions of very vigorous intensity activity

- a mix of moderate, vigorous and very vigorous intensity activity."[9]

· · • • • • • • · ·

It looks a lot when you see 150 minutes written in front of you, and the word 'vigorous' is a bit off-putting, but it's only two and a half hours spread over a whole week, or around 20 minutes a day, which could mean a brisk walk to the supermarket. Something is better than nothing, and you will make the most gains of all in terms of health by going from doing nothing at all to doing something.

It can seem a massive uphill struggle when starting from scratch with getting fitter. But in reality, it doesn't have to be complicated or hugely time-consuming. It's not like we're in the training montage from a *Rocky* film. Part of the problem is that fitness has become so commodified and over-analysed, that once you look into it, you will be told that you need to do yoga for flexibility, lift weights for strength, Pilates for core strength, running for cardiovascular health, cold water swimming for your immune system, HIIT training for weight loss, walking for mental health, and heaven knows what else. Oh, and did I mention, for best results you need to do each of them every morning before breakfast. It's only £8 a class, thank you very much.

It's just not possible.

If you want to run a marathon or compete in a strongman/woman competition, then clearly you have to put the hours in. But for the rest of us who just want to be 'fit enough', it's a good idea to look at it the other way around. How much time and effort are you willing and able to commit? There's no point signing up to run a marathon if you can only spare ten minutes a day. Throwing yourself in too hard and going from one extreme to another is not a good idea. Your body won't like it and it is unsustainable. It's much better to start by just doing a little more than you are already doing. And that 'bit more' might be enough anyway. There are things you can do in ten minutes that will improve your strength and flexibility. And there are probably ways you can sneak in a bit more movement at other times. There's no shame in starting small. If you hate the idea of exercise, why not just commit to ten minutes a day? It doesn't have to be all in one block, and those ten minutes will not be wasted time. In fact, they will do you a lot of good. And once you start to feel some benefits from the ten minutes, you might find you want to increase it to 12 minutes, or maybe 15. As Dr Rangan Chattergee says in his book, *Feel Better in Five: Your Daily Plan to Feel Great for Life*, if you spent five minutes a day chain-smoking cigarettes or solidly knocking back gin, it would have affect your body, so shouldn't we expect five minutes of doing something positive also to have an effect?

What might 150 minutes of exercise look like?

The recommended 150 minutes is supposed to be spread over an entire week and to be a mix of different types and intensity of exercise. This is on top of your normal daily movement.

Let's start with the recommendation to do strengthening activities on at least two days a week.

I am going to be deliberately non-prescriptive about what exercise you or I or anyone else ought to do on a weekly basis. Instead, we should look at moving our whole bodies as much as possible in as many ways as possible. (See chapter three for more ideas on this.) If you are looking for some ideas to get you started, there are some very simple exercises you can do that will build strength across your whole body.

Why start with strength training?

Strength is key. We condition men to think that they ought to be big and strong, and so lifting weights is something that many men will gravitate towards, but not so much for women. Which is strange when you think about what is traditionally seen as 'women's work'. Doing all the manual labour required to manage a house and family, all day, every day requires a huge amount of physical strength. Just carrying a baby around takes muscles, and then you probably would have to strap that baby to your back so you can work in the fields or cook meals. In traditional societies around the world, women need to be strong to dig the ground, carry water, do laundry and cleaning, grind and mash different seeds and vegetables, and be able to do all this while pregnant or with an infant in tow. This work is done by women and girls of all ages.

Physical strength is essential for everyone and is especially important for people as they get older. We don't want to end up getting frail, with weak and brittle bones. A bit of strength training is good for all of us.

How to get stronger

There's a good argument that if you can't lift your own bodyweight, why are you even thinking about pumping iron? Can you do a full press-up? You don't need any equipment to improve your strength using just the weight of your own body. This includes things like press-ups, planks, squats, and lunges. If you don't know how to do these, have a look at the exercises that trainers like Joe Wicks or Mr Motivator do. It's all stuff that can be done in a tiny space with no equipment. When you first get started pay very close attention to your form - if you are going it alone, look up something like 'proper form for a press-up' or 'proper form for a squat' to watch videos on how to do these movements in the safest way. Get someone to watch you, or film yourself, to see if you are doing it like the video.

Listen to your body when exercising. If anything hurts or feels wrong, stop.

When training to build strength, it is helpful to concentrate on the biggest muscles of the body, or as many muscle groups in one go as possible. You'll get the quickest, most noticeable results this way. Focus on your leg and bum muscles, as these are the big ones, and getting them stronger will make almost any other form of exercise easier.

In a few weeks, you will notice a difference if you do movements like this every day:

- Try doing squats and lunges whenever you are standing around waiting for the kettle to boil, or instead of bending to pick something up from the floor.

- Sit on the floor rather than on a chair. When you get up can you use just your legs—no hands?

Also, think about your core muscles, which are your abdominal muscles, pelvic floor and back muscles. These hold everything together and literally keep you upright. Core exercises could include:

- Standing on one leg. Do this any time you are standing around, for as long as you can. If this is easy, stand on a cushion to make the ground less stable. Can you do a minute on each leg?

- A daily plank. Time yourself and see if you can do 30 seconds.

- Anything from Pilates or Yoga.

Don't worry about anything more complicated than this. If you want to make a programme to follow, you could start by doing the following exercises one after the other:

1. Some squats

2. Some lunges

3. Some press ups (modified as necessary—search online for different options)

4. A plank

5. Hang from a bar (you can get pull-up bars that clip over a door frame. They are cheap and strong.)

You could do each one for 30 seconds using a timer app. That's it. Strength training done in two and a half minutes. You didn't need to get changed, use any equipment other than a pull-up bar, or go anywhere special. You could do that every day, right?

There are other ways of building strength that work just as well. Yoga builds strength, as does Pilates. Rock climbing is very much about using strength, especially in your upper back and forearms, plus core strength to keep your body close to the wall. Wrestling and Judo require strength. If you look at someone who does a lot of yoga or rock climbing, they won't look like your stereotypical image of a beefcake, but you can be strong without having big, bulging muscles. In fact, you want muscles that work through a range of motion, i.e. are flexible and useful, rather than puffed-up bodybuilder-type muscles.

What is moderate or vigorous exercise?

Moderate exercise gets your heart rate up, but you can still talk. This can include things like cycling, a brisk walk, maybe a game of football or a gentle jog. Dancing is moderate exercise (or vigorous if you're really going for it.)

Vigorous exercise is the stuff where your heart is pounding and you're out of breath. You are working about as hard as you possibly can. This could come from a game of squash, sprinting, or a HIIT session (high intensity interval training).

Let's say you do ten minutes of strength training three times a week, or maybe a single 30-minute yoga session. This is going to be moderate intensity if you're making sure that you work hard for those ten minutes. That leaves you with 120 minutes of your 150-minute total. If we spread that over six days of the week, you've got 20 minutes a day. Could you go for two ten-minute walks in a day? Maybe on a day off work you could go for a bike ride or play football with the kids or some friends for half an hour? You don't have to do the same routine every day, but it's important to be consistent in doing *something*.

It's easy to get overwhelmed by the choice of exercise and by feeling like you need to be setting aside hours and hours to do it. But what we've just seen is that it can be as simple as a ten-minute walk, a brief session of yoga, doing some squats and planks wherever you are, or whacking on some music for a kitchen disco.

I hate running. Do I have to run?

No! It is not necessary to run anywhere to get the health benefits of exercise and movement, or to get fitter. Running is a great form of exercise, with many positives, but it is not compulsory. Many fit people don't run. No one type of exercise is better than another.

The phrase, "don't run before you can walk" springs to mind. Walking is such a brilliant thing to do that it gets its own chapter later on. Never feel like an inferior exerciser because you walk rather than run.

You can build up your endurance in many ways, like swimming, tennis or cycling, as well as running or walking. What do you enjoy? What do your friends and family enjoy that you can do with them?

The advantage that running has over many other forms of exercise is that it gets you outside and you can go further than when walking in the same amount of time. It's great for your cardiovascular system and bone strength, and it's cheap. I don't have to get in my car and go anywhere to run, which means minimal excuses. I also feel like I've done a decent workout in just 20 minutes. It's also very accessible in that there are loads of running groups and clubs if you want to be sociable, and there are plenty of different apps that will help you train.

Learning how to run is a skill. It takes time to learn, and it takes time to go from finding jogging for 30 seconds challenging to being able to run a mile non-stop. Progress may feel slow, but following an app like *Couch to 5K* will build you up safely and relatively comfortably. Many people get into running almost by accident. They don't set out to become 'a runner', but find that they feel calmer and nicer after a run and actually look forward to it. I'm the first to say that I find running really hard and end up doing a lot of walking when I go out for a 'run'. But I have seen some beautiful sunrises on early morning runs. I've enjoyed jogging the dark streets at 5pm in December and nosing at everybody's Christmas decorations. I've experienced the camaraderie at Parkrun.[10] I have even enjoyed powering up a hill and feeling the strength in my legs as they carry me upwards. All of which could have been done at a walk too.

Exercise: not for nerds?

Many of us have grown up to believe that intellectual pursuits are more worthy than physical ones. British schools set us up with this belief from a young age, as the sitting and reading and writing activities quickly take over from the moving about and running around activities. P.E. gets squeezed out until it's a voluntary activity by the time you're in your mid-teens. As far as the education policymakers are concerned, it takes too much time away from the important business of learning Pythagoras' Theorem and how oxbow lakes are formed. We are expected to get as much knowledge into our heads as quickly as possible, and you need to sit still while you take it all in.

In the western world, we have a tradition of believing that the mind and body are separate entities, that they are made of different stuff, somehow. This means we believe we can have a mental life separate from our physical life. It stems back largely to Descartes and his "I think, therefore I am." It's the thinking thing, the mind, that is the only thing we can be sure of. After all, our bodies and the input from our senses can give us false information that we cannot rely upon to be true. We can hallucinate. Hormones and physical sensations can lead us astray. Our bodies are the vessels that carry us from place to place, but many prominent thinkers down the years have felt that the most worthy thing to do is lie around in bed and think important thoughts. (Which is not a bad thing.) Everything that we experience through our senses could be a lie; we could be plugged into the Matrix and not know it.

It's all part of our culture which values intellectual people over those who... aren't. Stephen Fry versus... how shall I put it? Gym bros. Meat heads. Air heads. Bimbos. They might be good fun, but not to be taken seriously. Perhaps they might even be considered a little vain? Frivolous? That's certainly not the case for all sports people, and there are plenty of insults that go the other way too: nerd, boffin, geek, etc. For those of us who fall squarely into the boffin and nerd category, the gym is not our natural habitat. It's a strange, testosterone-fuelled place, probably full of the people who bullied us at school. We don't feel like ourselves in sportswear, even if it comes in black.

What's all this got to do with getting fit? In an important respect, Descartes got it wrong. We cannot separate our mind from our body. The two are inextricably linked. The mind and body are one and the same. Your thoughts are very much affected by what's going on in your body, and vice versa. If you've got a terrible pain in your back, it's hard to think happy thoughts, or even to think anything at all that isn't related to how much your back bloody well hurts. What about the difference it makes to your mood, and your thoughts, when you have had a good night's sleep compared to a bad one? How well do you think when you're hungry? Our thoughts come from our physical experiences.

If we want our brains to function properly and work in the way they are supposed to, we need to move. Movement is the oil that lubricates the engine. One of the many good things it gives us is improved blood flow to the brain. This helps you think, and it helps your mood.

"Recent studies credibly have established that exercise stimulates the creation of new brain cells, pumps up existing ones, improves mood, aids in multitasking, blunts aging-related memory loss, sharpens decision making, dulls stress... and if you happen to be an elementary school student, improves your math grade."[11]

So if you're a nerd or a boffin, you'll be a much better nerd if you get some regular exercise. Going out for a walk or a jog, doing something that allows you to zone out, is great for helping your brain solve problems you are grappling with. Ancient Greek philosophers like Plato and Socrates, who even today we still look to for advice on how to live, firmly believed that exercise was vital for living your best life. Plato was a famous wrestler. He believed that being weak and weedy is no way to live and you won't be prepared for battle or anything else that life throws at you if you don't train your body alongside your mind.

Even if you have never thought that exercise is for you, you can enjoy all aspects of being in human form, and take joy from the physical as well as the cerebral. As the philosopher Damon Young says, in *How to Think About Exercise*, "there is an existential joy to workouts, which celebrates the whole human being."[12]

You don't have to choose between being Clark Kent and Superman. Be both!

Taking pleasure in exertion

We try to avoid unpleasantness and discomfort in our physical lives, and yet we sit for hours every day with mental dissatisfaction, whether that's stress at work or worrying about what's going on in the world. The delightful thing about exercise is that it allows us to shift the discomfort away from the mental and into the physical. You might think you've got enough unpleasantness in your life, so why would you want to add to it with exercise too? But if it's a discomfort of your own choosing you can control it and master it. While you are exercising you are temporarily distracted from the other worries you have. We rarely get satisfactory conclusions to problems in life, but overcoming a physical challenge is satisfying and rewards us with feelings of contentment and wellbeing.

We can take pleasure in exertion; it gives us a chance to achieve something we can celebrate. It doesn't matter how small that achievement is - if I have a session in the climbing gym where I climb a route I failed on last time, that's a win. I feel proud that I did that. It was entirely my own hard work; my strength and endurance and fearlessness got me to the top. Wins like that are not something we get too much of in daily life, when dealing with uncooperative children or colleagues, and working on projects that might take weeks to conclude. When we achieve something in an exercise or sporting context, it is more straightforward than in our ordinary lives. A win is a win.

Even if I don't succeed in my climbing project, there is still satisfaction to be gained from the effort. I know that every training session, every time I have a go at something, my body will get a little stronger and a little tougher. I am inching closer to what I want to achieve, even if the progress is slow and wonky. Every time I fail, I'm building my resilience, both physically and mentally. My body is learning how to recover and grow back stronger from setbacks and so is my mind.

Take pride in your body and what it can do. It's the only one you've got, and life is short, so make the most of it. Most of us won't get anywhere near the pinnacle of what our bodies are capable of - we don't have the time or inclination - but we can and should enjoy this aspect of ourselves. We can feel gratitude for whatever physical ability we have.

The rewards are worth it. A nice sit down after a long walk is a truly glorious feeling. It's a feeling of being tired out, but in a good way; physically tired but mentally alert and calm, with a feeling that you have earned a rest. An alien looking at people who have just finished a sports match or a hard workout might expect them to be miserable and exhausted. They have just put their bodies through what looks like a gruelling and painful experience. And yet, they are smiling! They look happy! What a difference from before the event. They are hugging each other and chatting, even with people they don't know. How can this be?

Just because 'the science' says so?

New scientific discoveries often tell us that something we previously thought was good is actually bad, and things we thought were bad are actually good. Look at skipping breakfast. When I was growing up in the 80s and 90s, breakfast was the most important meal of the day. We were told that people who skipped breakfast spent the rest of the day snacking on unhealthy foods and ended up fatter than people who ate a 'healthy' breakfast of cereal with milk and a glass of juice. Right? Wrong! Now we are told about the benefits of intermittent fasting, i.e. skipping breakfast. If you eat nothing for 14+ consecutive hours of the day, your body will repair and recover, your immune system will benefit, and they say you'll drop loads of weight because you can't ingest enough calories in the remaining 8 hours of the day to eat more than you would do at breakfast. (Although anyone with any history of eating disorders would be wise to steer well clear of this type of thing.)

If you believe what you read in the media, one week red wine is great for your health and the next week it's bad. The same goes for coffee, meat, or wheat. Running is both good for your knees and terrible for them. The fact is the facts change. All the stats about the benefits of exercise might look horribly antiquated in ten years' time. Maybe we'll look back and laugh at our naïve ideas. Often, studies on exercise are done on mice, rather than humans. And with humans it can be very difficult to do comprehensive studies on something like exercise that considers other variables like diet and genetics. Obviously, the scientists are aware of this, but just because 'studies' show x, y and z, doesn't mean that the results apply to you.

For example, I've tried skipping breakfast and I just can't do it. Maybe it's simply too hard for me to break a habit of a lifetime, but if I'm late for breakfast, I get shaky, woozy and I can't do anything at all. I need to eat in the morning. I've tried creeping breakfast later, but it doesn't work. Now, I know that if I couldn't have breakfast, I wouldn't actually die, but it's not something I can inflict upon myself—and I have tried. So even though 'the science' says it would be good for me to skip breakfast, I will not be taking them up on that suggestion.

Just as an aside, many of the scientific studies done on humans are actually done on young men, because women's bodies are too complicated with their pesky hormone cycles. For more on gender bias in science and medicine, I highly recommend that you read *Invisible Women*, by Caroline Criado Perez.

With exercise and fitness, I believe we should take an intuitive approach, rather than trying to incorporate all the recommendations from all the different studies. When you look at what 'the science' as a whole is telling us about exercise and movement, it's saying that doing some is good. All the health bodies around the world agree, and it's something people have been saying for literally thousands of years. It's unlikely to turn out to be wrong that being active is good for your health. It will benefit you now and in the long term. We don't need to concern ourselves with trying to do the very best or most scientifically recommended exercise possible - we're not athletes or looking to push the boundaries of peak human performance. Instead, we can focus on doing just enough. Don't become wedded to the idea that exercise has to look a certain way or that you have to do what everyone else is doing, or what is trendy right now. If you like the sound of something and it strikes a chord with you, give it a go.

·· • • •· • • •· ··

Remember:

- *Getting some exercise is vital for your physical health.*

- *It makes your immune system function better.*

- *It can improve sleep.*

- *Your mood can improve and it helps you cope better with stressful situations.*

- *Your chances of having a healthier old age improve.*

·· • • •· • • •· ··

Perhaps most importantly, I also find that feeling stronger and more robust gives me self-confidence. I know I am physically capable. I can lift a heavy thing and carry it somewhere. If I want to, I can walk a long way, or run, climb or swim. This makes me more open to new experiences and more likely to join in with other people doing fun things, because I know I can handle it. It's a vicious, or virtuous, circle: the less fit you are, the harder it feels to get fit, and the fitter you are, the more you feel the need to exercise. The trick is to start.

But hang on. So far, this is all so predictable, right? NHS guidelines, counting reps, going for a run... maybe there's another way to look at exercise?

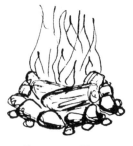

CHAPTER TWO

DID WE EVOLVE TO GO JOGGING?

How have we evolved to live?

We are too sedentary and it's making us ill. Our bodies are not working as they are supposed to because they are not getting enough movement.

When we are looking at how best to keep our bodies in good condition and to be fit to deal with what life throws at us, a good place to start would be to look at what we evolved to do. Four things in particular stand out:

1. Humans are social animals and moved together.

We have always lived in groups and relied heavily on the group for our survival. It's very hard to live completely on your own for any length of time if you've got to produce your own food, clothing, tools and shelter. Even if you had the skills to survive on your own, you would probably be pretty miserable. We don't do well alone. Recent studies on loneliness show that being lonely is worse for your health than smoking 15 cigarettes a day.[13]

In pre-industrial societies, work was done in a group. Women would gather food together, with grandmothers just as involved in the work or in looking after the babies. Men and boys would go hunting together. In ancient times, when predators abounded, it was also much safer to travel and work as a group. Lone humans with primitive weapons are pretty puny compared with a bear or a pack of wolves.

When agriculture was less mechanised, the whole village would be involved together in farming. Children would be expected to help with the harvest, which is why even today we have a long summer holiday from school. Cooperation and working with others were key to our survival.

2. People MOVED more. They had to.

As recently as last century, life was much more labour intensive than it is now. The invention of the automobile is incredibly recent in our history. It's only in the last one hundred years or so that people have had the possibility of owning a car, and it's even more recently that we have come to see it as normal for each adult in a household to have their own vehicle. Walking, riding a bicycle, taking public transport, riding a pony or using a horse and cart all require more movement than stepping out of your front door and plonking yourself straight into your car.

The further back you go, the more it becomes obvious just how much we would all have been moving about under our own steam. It is not just about the work required in tracking, catching, killing, skinning, gutting, preparing and cooking an animal before you eat it, it's also the activity required to gather the materials to make the fire, to make the tools, to build your own shelter, to pick plants or berries to eat with your roasted deer. There was an awful lot to do and it would take time. It wasn't all high intensity running about, it's hours of pottering and just being busy doing something.

By necessity, almost all work would require more physical activity than tapping away on a keyboard in front of a computer. People would have enjoyed a nice sit down, just as we do now, but even sitting or squatting uses more muscles if you don't have a chair with a back on it to hold you up or a table to rest your arms on. If you spend most your sitting time slouched on a sofa or supported by an office chair or car seat, all the work is done for you. Squatting is something we all would have done many times a day—it wasn't until relatively recently that toilets to sit on became widespread. Before then we would all have squatted, and in some cultures squat toilets are still the norm. If you don't regularly squat, see how hard it feels on your leg muscles to squat down and imagine holding yourself there to do a poo. Bet you didn't expect to be thinking about that today.

3. There was no processed food. All food required movement.

The 'Palaeolithic diet' has been a big hit over the last few years. In case you don't know what it is, the Paleo diet makes big claims about how slim and healthy we will be if we just eat the foods our ancestors would have eaten. From what I've seen, this often seems to revolve around a diet of steak, avocado, and bacon. The problem I have with this is that people seem to pick and choose the (expensive) foods they like best and justify them as being 'Paleo'. You can buy Paleo bars in the supermarket. But your cave dweller ancestors certainly couldn't pop to Tesco and buy a plastic wrapped 'Paleo bar'. If they lived anywhere other than South America they wouldn't have got their hands on an avocado either.

I don't think we realise just how easily attainable and convenient food has become. When my parents were children in the 1950s, you couldn't just go to your local fried chicken place and grab half a bird's worth of meat for a few quid and then eat it in the next ten minutes walking down the road. People never ate in the street or on public transport, and snacking wasn't a thing.

In the past, there would also have been more movement involved in preparing food. Without a food processor or blender there was chopping, mashing, and grinding to be done by hand. Meat would have been tougher when caught from the wild or allowed to grow at its normal rate, which means more chewing. Even something as simple as chewing is a form of movement that we have done away with in modern times!

4. Sitting down stress

Over the last few millennia, very little has changed in how human beings actually work. Our brains function in the same way our ancestors' brains did, and they work hard to protect us from danger and threats with exactly the same mechanisms they always used, whether you live in the jungles of Borneo or the urban jungle of London. Who's to say that chronic stress wasn't a thing for people in the past or in very different cultures? But we have a unique situation in the modern Western world that many people feel stressed all the time and have no physical relief or outlet for it.

When we are under stress, either through what's going on inside our heads or when we make demands of our bodies, we produce the hormone cortisol and a load of other chemicals. This is a very useful reaction because it is part of our natural 'fight or flight' mechanism and it happens within milliseconds of a trigger.

Producing cortisol is completely normal and something that happens as we wake in the morning or when we exercise. It gets us going. However, with chronic stress, if we produce too much cortisol for too long, in the worst-case scenario it can lead to increased blood sugar levels, weight gain, a suppressed immune system, digestive problems and heart disease. This is because cortisol inhibits insulin production and floods your muscles with glucose so that you have lots of energy for immediate use in fighting or running away. It also narrows the arteries and increases your heart rate, again so you're ready to deal with the threat. This is a perfectly rational response to a massive snarling wolf appearing on the path in front of you, but not so useful for dealing with that email from your boss. You don't want your blood sugar levels and your heart rate to be high unnecessarily.

The trouble is that our bodies just can't tell the difference between different types of threat. Whatever the perceived danger, our hormones only have the good old 'fight or flight' to deploy to deal with it. We aren't supposed to be in this state day in, day out. If the only dangers we faced were physical, then it would usually be over with fairly quickly, either because we died, or because we escaped to safety. Cortisol levels would spike and then return to normal when the danger passes. But because we are often dealing with stressful situations on a longer term or more chronic basis, we need to get the adrenaline and cortisol to calm the heck down. Stressful situations that are entirely sedentary would not have been a common human condition until recent times.

When you stop and think about how much movement people in the past would have been doing as part of normal life, just to survive, it's no wonder that our bodies and minds don't function particularly well on so little. We're starving ourselves with a lack of movement; we need it as much as we need nutritious food or sufficient sleep. The pace of change has been so rapid that in less than one hundred years we have designed out almost all movement from our lives. That's a blink of an eye in evolutionary terms.

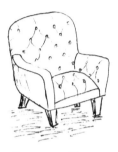

CHAPTER THREE

HOW DO I INCORPORATE MORE MOVEMENT INTO MY DAY?

Saving time costs us dearly

As we've seen, the guidelines about how much exercise we should do on a weekly basis don't say you have to do the lot in one go, or even in two or three chunks. In fact, it is much better for you to move frequently, rather than sitting on your backside all week and going for one mega run at the weekend. Our ancestors would have been active throughout the day, doing all the jobs that needed doing to feed the tribe. So the more often you can get up and move, the better.

"Even if you are physically active and fit, the more time you spend sitting in a chair, the higher your risk of chronic illnesses linked to inflammation, including some forms of cancer."[14]

If your normal day comprises going from bed to chair to car to chair to car to sofa to bed, your body is spending its entire time being supported by something. It barely has to work at all, as there is always a piece of furniture keeping you in position. You'll get weaker and weaker over time, and when you need to support yourself, your body will complain, making movement less appealing because it is HARD.

Basically, we all need to move as we did in the times before we had so many labour-saving devices. Machines save us effort, but have we gone too far in our desire for convenience? If you're up to date with your tech, you can control the music and lights in your house from your phone, so you don't even have to get up from your sofa because it's getting dark, or you want to change the radio station. Maybe you've got one of those doorbell cameras, so no more sprinting to answer the door in case it's that parcel you're waiting for. And on the subject of parcels, there's no need to trawl round the shops looking for the perfect pair of jeans. Just order a load online and send back the ones that don't fit. You'd think with all this convenience we must save so much time. But where is all that time we're saving? If you find it, let me know.

All these micro time savers add up to a lot of lost movement. If it's too late to stay lower tech in your home, you're going to have to get creative to add in the movement that we would have done without thinking 20 or 30 years ago, simply because we didn't have any choice. Having that choice has made moving so much harder.

Mix it up

We know that a varied diet of different foods is good for us, but what about a diet of varied movement?

Our modern lives are very unnatural. We are like animals in a zoo, constrained by hours of sitting and chronic stress. We rarely get to roam free. In Katy Bowman's excellent *Move Your DNA* she refers to diseases of captivity from which animals in zoos suffer. She gives the example of a killer whale endlessly circling a tiny tank - the whale's fin eventually becomes bent from always swimming around in a circle. She should travel for miles across the open ocean and when she lives in captivity her health suffers because she cannot move in the way she needs to.

We humans have also limited our own movement. Just because we have designed our own cages, doesn't mean it's not still a cage. We are subject to similar diseases of captivity as the killer whale in the circular tank. We don't get bent fins, but we do get humped backs and type-2 diabetes. Not only do we spend a lot of time sitting at a desk or on a comfy chair, those of us who do exercise often focus on just one thing, cycling or running, for example. These are great for our cardiovascular health, but can be a rather restricted set of motions. We'll strengthen up some areas at the expense of others. There are some complaints in the sedentary world that come up time and again, such as tightness in the hips, painful neck and shoulders, lower back issues. Most of the time, these problems are caused by how we spend most our days - the odd half an hour of exercise will not do much to counteract the many hours we spend in a limited number of positions. It's not that these positions are wrong, per se, but we're not designed to spend as much time in them as we do. It's not wrong to sit at a desk, but if that's all you do all day long, it's likely to lead to some painful problems. How we spend most of our time is going to influence the shape of our bodies.

For us quitters, we don't need to worry too much about over-training one set of muscles. We will not be doing enough cycling to develop Chris Hoy's thighs, for example. But we can be aware that when thinking about how to move and what to do, aiming for a variety of different things in frequent bouts is going to benefit our muscles and joints, and help undo some of the detrimental effects of limited movement in the rest of our daily lives. It's also great news for those of us who find repetitive exercise mind-numbingly boring.

This is where activities such as gardening or playing with children can be really useful, as they are varied and get you moving all of your body parts. If you have neither a garden/allotment or child, then consider other ways to move that use your whole body as you go about your daily business. Notice when you have been sitting for an hour or more. How many of your body parts have you actually moved today? Have you done any twisting, turning, bending, reaching up, squatting down?

If we can move our bodies in our daily activities that require using our muscles, we will soon find that we are doing enough to meet the guidelines. Add in two 10-minute brisk walks on top and you won't need to worry about doing traditional daily "exercise" at all. The challenge is getting your muscles working as part of your normal day.

Ideas to move more

Here are some simple ideas for adding more movement into your day. Just focus on whatever appeals to you. This isn't an exhaustive list, and I am sure you will have some of your own. Become more aware of when you are sedentary or times you might be taking the easy option or avoiding movement. Here are some ideas you could try:

Balance on one leg, one minute on each side, while cleaning your teeth. Balancing on one leg is superb for your core strength. If it's too easy for you, try doing it with your eyes closed...

Do a slow-as-you-can squat while cleaning your teeth or waiting for the kettle to boil. This is fantastic for your leg strength. If you can make a squat last a whole minute, i.e. 30 seconds to go down and 30 seconds to come back up again, you'll certainly feel it.

Dance! Put your favourite tunes on in the kitchen while cooking or doing chores. The crazier and more vigorous the dance moves the better, especially with someone else you can have a laugh with.

Muck about with the kids (yours or a friend's). Kids love rough and tumble play, and it's fantastic for their development and your bond. This is the ultimate long-term strength training too, because over time they get bigger and heavier and if you can still throw them up in the air when they are eight years old, you know you've got stronger. If you have grown up kids, look forward to moving on to rough and tumble play with the grandkids instead.

Run up the stairs—and be less efficient. You know how you go into another room to get something and realise you forgot the thing you needed, so you have to go back again? Embrace this. Why make one trip when you can make multiple trips at double the speed?

Squat to pick things up, e.g. while hanging up washing. Don't just bend down, squat! I did this while putting away the clean laundry last night. I squatted down to pick up every item from the basket. It was great exercise and gave my muscles a load of extra movement that they wouldn't have got otherwise, in no more time than I would have normally spent on that chore.

Install a pull-up bar over a door frame. Hang for as long as you can every time you go through that door. Few of us can actually do a pull-up, but working on your grip strength by hanging is extremely useful.

Put the things you need in more awkward places. We put the things we use most in the place that's at the easiest height. What if you put things higher up, or lower down, so you have to stretch or bend/squat to get to them? So what if no one who visits your house can find the teaspoons because you've put them in the very bottom drawer?

Spend ten minutes doing stretches in the evening. You can do this every day. Put on some nice relaxing music or just do it in front of the TV. When you turn on the TV, instead of sitting down, do some stretches while watching. Maybe keep the remote away from the sofa. If you have to move to get it, you could do some stretches while you're about it.

Make your own bread. Kneading bread dough for ten minutes is an excellent arm workout. The rest of the bread-making process doesn't take much longer than this. You mix up the dough, knead it for ten minutes, leave it in a warm place for a couple of hours, or until you realise you've forgotten all about it. Another quick knead, stick it in a tin, forget about it again, then bake (ideally when you've already got the oven on for something else). You then get to eat the bread! There are other ways to incorporate movement into preparing food, such as whisking or mixing by hand. You could look back in the history of your food culture and recreate what your great-grandmother would have been making.

Sit on the floor. Instead of always heading straight for the sofa, try sitting on a cushion on the floor. You will find that you naturally move around a lot more (because it's less comfortable!) There are many positions you can sit or lie in. You have to use your muscles to support yourself to stay upright, and it also takes more muscles to get up and down. Can you get up from the floor without using your hands? Several movement specialists I know are so convinced of the benefits of sitting on the floor that they have removed all the furniture from their houses. They sit or squat on the floor all the time, including for meals, using low coffee tables to put their food on. They also eschew comfy beds. I mean, it is how our ancestors would have lived...

Park further away from the shops. Always choose to walk whenever possible. It's such an old chestnut, isn't it? Take the stairs rather than the lift, park at the far end of the car park. You've heard it all before. It adds up though—think about the strength you're gaining in your leg muscles from walking or running up the stairs. That's 'proper' exercise that people pay for the privilege of doing at a gym. If it's less than half an hour's walk away, and you feel safe in the area, do you really need to drive or get public transport?

Make a walk with a friend one of your social activities. Honestly, you will have the best chats walking side by side with someone. You'll walk for longer and it'll feel much easier than going alone.

See the benefits of doing the housework. Get scrubbing! I find cleaning, especially vacuuming, is hard, physical work. I hate it. Getting it over and done with as quickly as possible gets me out of breath and in a sweat, so it definitely counts as exercise.

Fidget. People who fidget a lot can burn off an extra 300 calories a day. You can set an alert on your phone to tell you to move every hour if you have a tendency to sit in one place for too long.

Get a watch with a step counter. See what you do on a normal day and challenge yourself to increase it. Mine works out my average steps and then encourages me to try to achieve this every day. There is more on counting steps in chapter five.

If you go to the gym, make sure your gym bag is always ready by the door. That way, it's always there if you're in a hurry. I've heard of people going to sleep in their gym gear so they can get straight up and go for a run in the morning. This might be extreme, but make sure any equipment or clothing you need is easily accessible, preferably in line of sight.

When waiting for something or someone, pace about. A friend told me that when her son is at swimming lessons, instead of sitting with the other parents, she puts a podcast on her headphones and walks around. Another friend walks around the football pitch when her daughter is training.

Make your mobile immobile. When you're at home, leave your mobile phone in one place so that you have to go to it when you want to use it.

Pay attention to how you talk to yourself: change your language to say to yourself, "How am I going to move today?" Make it non-negotiable in your head. Being disciplined is hard. If you are a person who likes lists, add it to your to-do list. Instead of "I might do some yoga later if I have time", it needs to be, "when am I going to do my yoga?" and fit it into your plan for the day. As we've seen, it's not rational to want to waste energy on exercise and I find it's the first thing I drop if I'm pushed for time. There's a lot more about motivation in the second half of this book.

It's difficult to find the time to exercise, and it can also appear that by making tasks take longer, for example by walking somewhere instead of driving, that this leaves even less time in the day. But by combining daily tasks with movement, you are actually getting twice as much done. The more we can add movement to the things we already do, the less additional time we have to find to do movement or exercise as a standalone activity.

Be curious and keep an open mind about new and unusual ways to move more of your body more often.

Clothes

What you wear affects how you move. Whatever your gender, if you have ever worn high heels, a tight skirt and a corset you'll know that you move very differently when dressed like this from when you're wearing a tracksuit. While it may feel great to dress up sometimes, if you are looking to increase your movement, what you wear will affect your success. Wearing tight, restrictive clothing won't help you do a few squats while hanging up the washing, or to have a stretch while the kettle's boiling. Pencil skirts are no good when you want to run up the stairs. Even if you have to look smart for your job, there are plenty of options for both men and women's clothing that have a bit of stretch in (unless it's a uniform of course).

Because I am always looking for an excuse, I find if I have to get changed to do exercise, I mentally factor in how much time it's going to take me and then decide I haven't got time. It's completely illogical, but I would rather go for an hour's walk in clothes I'm already wearing than a 20-minute run, which, including getting changed and a quick shower, would also take an hour. Basically, I will exploit any perceived barrier, no matter how small, and use it as an excuse not to exercise. So it's a good idea to wear clothes every day that you can do most types of movement in without having to change into something special.

While on the subject of clothing, there are two ways to go when deciding what to wear to exercise in. Firstly, it really doesn't matter what you wear, as long as it's comfortable and appropriate for the conditions. You don't have to wear sports leggings and a tight vest top to go for a run. Many of us prefer something baggier. If you want to go for a bike ride in chinos and a shirt, and they are stretchy and comfy, then why not? If you're exercising at home, pyjamas are fine, there's no need to get changed. It's not like you're a professional cyclist looking to shave milliseconds off your time by wearing skintight Lycra. Better just to get on and do it, rather than faff about for ages getting changed.

Secondly, you might also find it encouraging to get yourself some nice clothes for exercising in. If how you look is important to you and you don't want to jog the streets looking like you've just crawled out of bed, then a bit of shopping can be an excellent incentive.

Shoes

Comfortable shoes are a must, and the flatter the sole, the better. Even the smallest heel affects the shape of your leg, which forces your muscles to work differently to their natural design. Imagine walking down a hill, and how being at that angle pulls on your quads on the front of your thighs, and puts pressure on your knees. Even the smallest raise on the heel of your shoe is like always walking slightly downhill. Very often, back, hip and knee problems can be traced back to your feet. The way you walk and the angle of your feet can lead to stresses and strains much further up your body as it compensates for an imbalance down at the bottom.

Shoes are a relatively recent invention, especially shoes with a raised heel. They were useful for keeping your foot in a stirrup when riding a horse, and nowadays they are considered attractive for women because wearing heels pushes your bum up and out, but they are not helpful for getting you to move in the most comfortable and efficient way. Even trainers, which we think of as flat and comfy, often are significantly higher at the heel than the toe. Some trainers effectively have a 1-inch heel on them. Instead, look for the flattest shoes you can. In technical terms, you may see them called 'zero drop', 'minimal' or 'barefoot' footwear.

It's also a good idea to look for shoes that have plenty of space for your toes to splay, so your feet can move how they are supposed to. Just like your hands don't work so well in a mitten, your feet don't work at their best when compressed within a shoe. If your toes can spread, the muscles in your feet can work properly and they will get stronger. Having strong and flexible feet will allow you to move easily over different terrain and your foot will bend and stretch to accommodate bumpy ground. This is great for improving your balance, which is vital as we age. If your feet aren't able to do their job because they are cocooned by thick, rigid shoes, then your other joints and muscles higher up will have to work harder than they should, which again, isn't great news for your knees or hips.

We take in a lot of sensory information through the soles of our feet. By wearing shoes with thin soles (or no soles at all) our feet can tell our brains what the surface underfoot is like. If you can't remember ever walking barefoot on grass, try it. I love walking over cobblestones in thin-soled shoes. It feels wonderful to be so connected to the earth, rather than being separated from it by a thick layer of plastic.

Making the switch to shoes with less heel and padding can feel strange at first, and initially your feet might feel tired after wearing them, but after a while your muscles will toughen up and I promise you, you won't want to go back to chunky, narrow, restrictive footwear. Start with short walks and build up slowly because your calf muscles will be working harder than they used to—they will have to stretch further than before to get your heel to the ground.

I do most of my walking in barefoot-style shoes, but I don't run in them because I need a bit of cushioning on the pavements. If you are serious about getting into running, then there are many options for the shape of the sole, and a specialist sports shoe shop will help you find the most comfortable pair for you. It's worth trying on a few different styles, as the differences between them can be huge. If you are interested in barefoot running, have a look online at how to do it. It's not as simple as just changing your shoes.

I must say that barefoot shoes are not cheap, but the range of shoes available is getting better all the time, so I hope that they will get cheaper. Plimsoll- or Converse-style shoes also have thin, flat soles, so as long as they aren't too narrow in the toe, these can be a great, cheap option for the summer months. Also, sandals can have nice flat soles. Just make sure you have a strap round the heel—flip flops and sliders are terrible to walk in because you have to clutch them with your toes to hold them onto your foot. You can also try beach shoes/swimming shoes, which are very cheap.

If you want to buy new shoes but can't stretch to the £70 - £150 for most barefoot shoes—ironic that something 'minimal' is so expensive—then look for the flattest heel possible and a nice wide toe area.

Even though I'm evangelical about them, I realise barefoot shoes aren't for everyone. At least aim to wear shoes that have flexible soles so your feet can flex and curve around uneven terrain. If your feet are comfy and working properly it will help encourage you to move.

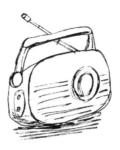

CHAPTER FOUR

DANCE

Something that struck me when I was researching this book was how dance is such an integral part of every culture around the world. Think of any group of people, anywhere in the world, and you'll find a traditional dance. People dance as a welcome, a farewell, a celebration, to appease the gods, to let off steam. It comes naturally to us.

Dances can last for hours or even days. From an all-night rave in a field in Essex, to the nine-night Navratri festival in Gujarat, India, we dance and dance and dance. We bond and communicate through dance and even love watching other people dancing.

Dancing doesn't feel like exercise. If you're looking for a way to get your heart rate up that is genuinely fun–not 'fun' like fitness trainers say a session of circuit training is 'fun'–then dance is it.

I've talked about taking pleasure in exertion, and dancing is probably the ultimate expression of this. When was the last time you lost yourself in dancing to music?

I used to dance for hours in nightclubs. I must have burned off thousands of calories at sweaty rock nights, followed by a trek home up one of Bristol's steep hills. Cider and chips were my fuel of choice in those days. Twenty years later and I rarely dance, partly because of a lack of nightlife and probably also because I don't drink as much cider, being old and sensible.

In contrast to my moshing days, I used to dance around a lot more gently when my kids were very young. I'd sway from side to side, even when in the queue at the supermarket on my own, as I was so used to constant movement to calm a fractious baby. Parents instinctively sing and dance with their babies and toddlers as much of our learning happens through linking movement to rhythm. We teach babies and children counting and other concepts like naming their body parts through songs and movements. It's the way we learn about proprioception, or where your body is in space. I bet you can remember *Heads, Shoulders, Knees and Toes*, or *The Macarena*, even if you haven't heard either of them for decades. Our bodies and brains respond particularly well to moving to music. We do songs with actions like *Row, Row, Row Your Boat* because small children love to move to music. It's a timeless ritual: we sing the same songs to our babies that were sung to us when we were small. I hope my children sing *Row, Row, Row Your Boat* to their own babies one day. They might sing *Baby Shark*, I suppose. I don't know the moves to that one.

Watching a toddler dance is one of life's most joyful experiences. Joining in is even better. Their bopping around isn't even in time with the music, but it is full of the passion for life and self-love that small children possess. Forget 'dance like nobody's watching', I prefer to 'dance like a toddler'.

It doesn't matter how you dance or what type of music you dance to. You can dance by yourself or with a partner. You can do classes and structured routines, or go free form and make it up as you go along. Do the twist, the macarena, or the hokey cokey. Slow or fast. Embrace your inner raver or your inner toddler.

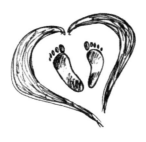

CHAPTER FIVE

SLOW AND STEADY FOR THE WIN: WHY WALKING IS THE BEST

What's not to like?

If you are looking for easy ways to get more movement into your life, the best thing to do is walk.

Walking is what humans are good at. Compared with most other animals, our bodies are really efficient at walking long distances. If we're in good condition, we can walk for hours, no problem.

I must confess that I am biased in writing this chapter because I love walking and can honestly say it was my saviour through the pandemic. It gave me space away from the house. Walking with a friend was my only form of in-person socialising, plus it kept me fit. I've always felt a connection with walking anyway, but the lockdowns exaggerated it.

It's not just me though, just look at how many books are about long walks, either about the journey itself, the people and places visited on the way, or about the epiphanies experienced by the walker. The Romantic poets were very keen on a walk: "I *wandered lonely as a cloud*," and all that.

Don't feel you have to be going on massive hikes all the time. The NHS says:

> "You do not have to walk for hours. A brisk 10-minute daily walk has lots of health benefits and counts towards your recommended 150 minutes of weekly exercise."[15]

What's not to like about going for a walk? You don't need any special equipment, just comfortable shoes and weather-appropriate clothing. You don't have to sign up to anything, measure anything, or pay for anything. And it's something you can incorporate into your daily activities pretty easily. Whether you live in a town or village, there's bound to be a little job you can do which can involve ten minutes of walking, whether that's posting a letter (old school, I know) or going shopping. You can walk to a pub or a café. As long as you can physically walk, walking is a form of movement you can fit in around anything else you're doing.

The ancient philosopher Diogenes coined the phrase s*olvitur ambulando*, meaning "it is solved by walking". Time spent walking is time to think, to ponder, to breathe, to have uninterrupted time to talk with a loved one. Walking encourages creative thought. Ideas spring forth when they had previously been trapped behind the confines of a desk.

> "Busy with pounding legs and pumping arms, the intellect's walls come down, and previously parted ideas and impressions can freely mingle..."[16]

Whether or not you think walking will solve your problems, you might approve of this Noel Coward quote:

> "I like long walks, especially when they're taken by people I dislike."

The health benefits of walking

For most of us, walking is an easy form of exercise. Is it too easy to be as good for us as running, swimming, or CrossFit? Don't be fooled into thinking that hardcore exercise is necessarily preferable. You can get more than enough good stuff from the simple act of putting one foot in front of the other. For thousands of years, people have known that walking is good for you. Hippocrates, the 'father of medicine', who lived 2,400 years ago, believed no medicine has as broad an effect as going for a walk. As usual in our culture, we don't believe it until some scientists have done their research, and funnily enough, they agree with Hippocrates, as we instinctively knew they would.

·· • • •·• • ··

The benefits of walking include:

- *Improved cardiovascular health*

- *Stronger bones and joints*

- *Increased longevity*

- *Helping to reduce insomnia, especially with a morning walk*

- *Lower Alzheimer's risk*

- *Improved mood*

- *Strengthened muscles*

- *Increased support for joints*

- *Slower mental decline*

·· • • •·• • ··

The list of benefits of walking goes on and on. This is from Harvard Health, the consumer health education division of Harvard Medical School, 10th June 2021:

> **"It counteracts the effects of weight-promoting genes.** Harvard researchers looked at 32 obesity-promoting genes in over 12,000 people to determine how much these genes actually contribute to body weight. They then discovered that, among the study participants who walked briskly for about an hour a day, the effects of those genes were cut in half.

> **It helps tame a sweet tooth.** A pair of studies from the University of Exeter found that a 15-minute walk can curb cravings for chocolate and even reduce the amount of chocolate you eat in stressful situations. And the latest research confirms that walking can reduce cravings and intake of a variety of sugary snacks.

> **It reduces the risk of developing breast cancer.** Researchers already know that

any kind of physical activity blunts the risk of breast cancer. But an American Cancer Society study that zeroed in on walking found that women who walked seven or more hours a week had a 14% lower risk of breast cancer than those who walked three hours or fewer per week. And walking provided this protection even for the women with breast cancer risk factors, such as being overweight or using supplemental hormones.

It eases joint pain. Several studies have found that walking reduces arthritis-related pain, and that walking five to six miles a week can even prevent arthritis from forming. Walking protects the joints — especially the knees and hips, which are most susceptible to osteoarthritis — by lubricating them and strengthening the muscles that support them.

It boosts immune function. Walking can help protect you during cold and flu season. A study of over 1,000 men and women found that those who walked at least 20 minutes a day, at least five days a week, had 43% fewer sick days than those who exercised once a week or less. And if they got sick, it was for a shorter duration, and their symptoms were milder."[17]

You might think you haven't got time to walk every day. It's funny isn't it, how people will find the time to walk a dog because the dog *needs* to be walked every day, when really, it's us who need the daily walk.

I would walk ten thousand steps and I would walk ten thousand more

It has become part of our general knowledge that we ought to do 10,000 steps a day. That's around five miles, depending on the length of your stride. Phones and smartwatches have step counters, so it's quite easy to track, though they often aren't very accurate. The definition of 'sedentary' is anything below the threshold of 5,000 steps per day, so it's worth tracking your number of steps to get an idea of how much you really are moving every day.

If you manage 10,000 steps in a day, it shows that you have been pretty active, whether it's because you've been for a decent walk or run, or you have been on your feet a lot throughout the day. The target includes both exercise and your daily general movement. But do we really need to aim for 10,000 steps? Where did that target come from?

It's not a target that has any sort of historic basis, as adults in modern hunter-gatherer societies take around 20,000 steps per day, which equates to around nine miles.[18]

20,000 steps a day is unrealistic for most of us. It's hard to find the time, let alone the enthusiasm, to walk ten miles a day. In fact, the average Brit or American manages barely a quarter of this. However, the 10,000 target came originally from a Japanese manufacturer of a pedometer in the 1960s. They chose the name *Manpo-kei*, which means "ten-thousand-step meter", because they liked the sound of it. So it was an arbitrary, made up target that just caught on. But what is the latest thinking from the scientists studying this stuff?

A recently published study suggests that middle-aged people doing at least 7,000 steps a day had a 50%-70% reduced risk of mortality.[19] Taking over 10,000 steps per day was not found to have any further reduction in mortality risk. However, as is often the case, the study has its limitations:

> "The lowest step group had the highest rates of cardiovascular disease, hypertension, and diabetes. Although our analyses attempted to control for these and other health status factors,

there remains potential for residual confounding and reverse causality."[20]

The scientists found it hard to draw conclusions to suggest that the people who do more steps are healthier *because* of the steps, rather than because they don't already have pre-existing conditions which mean they physically can't do over 7,000 steps a day. Having said that, this isn't the only study showing that more steps per day are beneficial, and you can use counting steps as a good indicator to see how active you are. Can you do 7,000 steps in a day?

However, rather than focusing too heavily on a number, the current advice seems to be more concerned with the briskness of the walk:

> "Just 10 minutes of brisk walking a day is an easy way for adults to introduce more moderate intensity physical activity into their day and reduce their risk of early death by up to 15%."[21]

This makes sense, because by going a little faster, you'll get your heart rate up and your muscles will have to work harder. This is what will put walking into the 'moderate intensity' bracket. If you find brisk walking tough, try listening to upbeat music - there are various playlists available that have music with the beats-per-minute you need. The guidance is that if you want to get fitter, you ought to aim for a pace of 100 steps-per-minute. Depending on your current level of ability at walking, this might feel too fast or too slow. If you want to get fitter, simply walk faster than you currently do. Katy Bowman has some suggestions for you to pace yourself with, so you don't have to try to count while walking:

> "Measuring your steps-per-minute is pretty freaking boring. A fun way to challenge your pacing is to use a song's beats-per-minute (bpm) as your stepping-rate guide. Beyonce's "Crazy in Love" and Stevie Wonder's "Superstition" are 100bpm. You can try some 120bpm for comparison: "I Wanna Dance With Somebody" by Whitney Houston, "Enter Sandman" by Metallica, "Don't Stop Believin'" by Journey. You can check your pace by humming a few bars to see how your steps measure out."[22]

A quick internet search will come up with various songs and playlists at 100 bpm. I find I walk faster when on my own than with a friend, and even faster when listening to upbeat music. It's difficult not to step in time with the beat. Try putting headphones on next time you walk somewhere. Use music to help you: you will go faster and further.

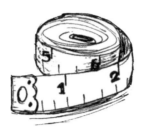

Chapter Six

Can I Exercise Myself Slim?

For most of human history, and in large parts of the world today, getting enough food to survive is the issue. Not starving to death is the primary worry around food. However, in countries like the UK, we're now in the unusual position of many of us having too much food, too easily available. People in the West have got taller and fatter over the last few generations, and we continue to get fatter. In 2019, it was estimated that 64% of people in the UK were overweight or obese.[23] Carrying a bit of excess weight probably won't cause any health issues in most of us, but the problem is that it *feels* like an issue. It's making us miserable. Many of us, myself included, have seen exercise as a route to losing weight, and probably the only reason we'll force ourselves into joining a gym or taking a class is because we think it's going to make us thin. If you're reading this book hoping by moving more you'll get slimmer, read on.

There is a lot of pro-exercise lobbying from food manufacturers who suggest that you can eat their chocolate bars or drink their fizzy drinks and stay slim as long as you do lots of exercise. Or the fact that there are always junk food vending machines at the swimming pool or gym. These snacks and drinks are packed with sugar, and the manufacturers get away with it because they promise that it's exercise, not diet, that will make you slim. We buy into this myth because we like the taste of the foods and because we mistakenly believe that exercise burns more calories than it actually does.

Don't shoot the messenger, but I'm sorry to say that you probably won't lose weight by exercise alone. Not everyone agrees on this, but the general thinking seems to be that healthy eating is the most effective way to lose or control weight, with exercise playing a helpful role in maintaining weight loss.[24] We burn off fewer calories than we might think by exercising, and our bodies compensate for the calories burned by moving less or eating a bit more afterwards, without us realising what we're doing. If you want to lose weight, the first place to look is to your fridge, rather than to your sportswear. That doesn't mean we shouldn't try to move more; aside from all the health benefits, regular exercise such as strength training will make you look better from having greater lean muscle mass, even if your scales don't read any differently. If you do lose weight, exercise is really useful in helping you to maintain the weight loss.

So controlling our food intake is the way to go. But dieting is hard. Does going on a diet work actually any better than trying to do more exercise?

Diets are big business, with the diet industry being worth an estimated £2bn a year. You cannot avoid being exposed to weight loss marketing from companies, campaigns by the government and, if you are overweight, pressure from health professionals, even if you have gone to see them for something completely unrelated. But we are all still getting fatter. The pressure isn't working. The diet industry doesn't appear to be helping people to lose weight and keep it off.

Why diet plans don't work

My social media feeds bombard me with adverts from diet companies, each promising a more scientific approach than the last. They will "use science", "reset my hormones", or best of all, get the weight to fall off me with seemingly no effort or food restriction on my part. The most insidious ones seem to me like cults, where they use real people to sell their products for them. I've got a couple of friends who have joined one of these groups. Every other post is about how amazing they feel, with pictures of how slim they are now, clutching strange looking teas and shakes in plastic bottles. After a few of these posts, one pops up saying they are looking for fellow 'ladies' to join them in their amazing healthy plan. It's a pyramid scheme. They are looking for recruits to sell more shakes and teas to. It's a business. The shakes and teas are made in bulk somewhere. Someone is making a big profit off getting my friends to flog their powders for them.

If a diet company sells food or food replacement products - shakes, bars, or 'meals' - is it really in their interest that their 'quick fix' works long term? Or do they make more profit if you have some success and reach your goal, but as soon as you go off the plan you regain the weight, meaning you come back to them for more? The shareholders need you to keep buying their products. Pre-made diet foods like milkshakes and ready meals may be convenient, but they are also anti-social and expensive. If you are cooking for a family, you're going to be making something separate for yourself, which might be fine for a while but is probably unsustainable if your special diet food is more expensive and less satisfying than what you're feeding everyone else.

When trying out one of these plans, you need to consider the end game. You will not be able to sustain this for the rest of your life, so you need to decide what you are going to do when you have lost the weight you want to lose. And don't forget, your body will be very keen for you to regain that weight, or at least some of it.

Lots of these diets sell themselves as a lifestyle that's so easy. But if that's the case, why do people stop the diet and regain the weight?

Studies have shown that only around 20% of dieters (who lose 10% of their bodyweight) maintain that weight loss for more than a year. Important factors in maintaining the weight loss were keeping up with the healthy eating and exercising, but also being able to regulate emotions and having lower levels of depression.[25]

Fat people are some of the most stigmatised in our society. It seems to be socially acceptable to discriminate against someone who is bigger, because people think it's a choice to be fat, which is absolute rubbish. Does anyone actively choose to be overweight?

There are sometimes health reasons why someone might be overweight. Maybe they are on medication that makes them more liable to put on weight. However, let's not forget that emotional causes of weight gain are just as valid.

I would guess that most us have a complicated relationship with food and exercise, stemming from what we experienced at home growing up, and what we experienced in school. Body image issues come from several places, but what we heard from our parents or carers as children is key. Did you see your mother always on a diet? Were you made to feel that looking a certain way was essential to be popular, or even loved?

As a society, we are aware of mental health now more than ever. Yet that understanding and kindness doesn't seem to trickle through into acceptance of people's inability to exercise or their compulsion to overeat or eat unhealthy foods.

People who suffered abuse as children are more likely to become overweight adults, especially women who suffered sexual abuse. An abusive childhood is also more likely to lead to ill health generally later in life, and this ill health can also be an indirect cause of weight gain. Let's have a bit of compassion, shall we?

At the same time, were you taught how to cook healthy, nutritious food? Were you brought up to feel like certain foods or drinks were 'naughty' or a treat? Something to reward yourself with after a hard day, or to cheer you up when you're sad? Do you *need* chocolate or alcohol to relax? I think all of us can look back into our past and see where we might have got certain hang-ups or issues with food. Many of us turn to food as a comfort, to help us deal with negative emotions, because we weren't shown any other way. If you're happy, celebrate with an enormous special meal. If you're sad, drown your sorrows with wine or eat your way through it with chocolate or crisps. If you're rushed off your feet, just grab something quick and tasty, which usually means wrapped in plastic, highly processed and full of sugar. It's no wonder so many of us are overweight.

If we only ate when we were truly hungry, and stopped the second we were full, we wouldn't struggle nearly so much with our weight. This kind of intuitive eating is what children do naturally—if we don't tempt them with sweets and chocolate—and is what most animals do. Clearly it is too easy to get hold of high calorie, delicious food that is very difficult to resist. There are a few people around who only see food as fuel and would be happy to get all their nutritional needs from a pill, but most of us derive enormous pleasure from food.

The factor that I think often gets missed in conversations about diet is why we overeat in the first place, and what is making us all eat too much of the wrong things. There is a massive emotional component to eating, which makes us turn to the very foods that are most likely to make us gain weight.

Not having an emotional attachment to eating would make a massive difference to our eating habits. If you feel you eat too much when you don't need to, have a think about the following:

· · • • • • • • · ·

Why do you eat, other than being hungry?
Is it:

- *The time of day? It's 1pm, therefore it is time to have lunch.*

- *Because you're doing something else like watching a film and are mindlessly popping chocolates into your mouth?*

- Social pressure? *The people around you encourage you to eat more than you need.*

- *Because you're tired and need the energy?*

- *Because you're bored, fed up or sad and need cheering up?*

- *Because you're stressed?*

········

The first two on the list are really about mindless eating and eating out of habit. The others are more about emotions. Until we become aware that we are eating for reasons other than hunger, and choosing foods to meet our emotional needs, we don't have a hope of changing what we eat. Your emotions will nearly always override what you know you ought to do. Food is comforting. Milk is comforting to babies, and most of us never really grow out of that need to use food in this way. Couple that with the high stress society we live in, and it's no wonder at all that many of us help our emotions with nice food.

As an example, I'd like to introduce you to my cat, Lionel, who as I write this is standing next to my keyboard, head-butting me for attention.

When we brought home Lionel from a rescue centre in May 2017, he had been stuck in there for a few months. Imprisoned, Lionel would say. He ate anything and everything you put in front of him. If you put down a bowl of cat biscuits, he would eat the lot in one go, rather than picking at them now and then like most cats I've known. The people at the rescue centre would give him all the other cats' leftovers and he would hoover them up. When he came to live with us, he would lie on my chest first thing in the morning and he was so heavy I could barely breathe, which was a very effective tactic to get me out of bed so I could feed him.

Once he got used to living with us, and realised that he would not be sent to live in a pen again, his eating became normal. While I can't exactly say he's svelte (small children can't lift him) he has definitely slimmed down. He will leave food if he doesn't like it, and he has decided that he only likes expensive cat food. No supermarket own-brand for our Lionel.

For Lionel, the stress of being in an unnatural environment, where he had no control over where he went or what he did, led to him overeating. Being in a difficult situation meant he reacted perfectly sensibly. After all, if you are unsure of your environment, you can't trust where the next meal is going to come from, so it makes sense to eat everything while you can. You're protecting yourself by getting as many calories in as possible. It took time for him to realise that he was 'home' but luckily for him, when he did, he could relax and eat normally again. If the stress had carried on, he would probably have continued overeating.

There is no quick fix to emotional eating. No quick fix diet is going to solve the root cause of the problem. We overeat and choose high fat, high sugar foods because we are stressed or sad. This can be because we feel bad and sad about things outside of ourselves, the circumstances we find ourselves in, or it can be because we feel bad and sad about ourselves. If you look in the mirror and hate what you see, maybe it'll spur you onto a diet where you can further punish yourself by cutting out all the things that give you a bit of joy in life, or you might go the other way and comfort yourself for feeling awful by eating and drinking things which will give you a moment's respite from the self-loathing. Sugary, fatty foods feel nice in the mouth and give you a hit of energy that no amount of cucumber is going to provide.

There may be other, deeper emotional issues at play here too, which stem from childhood experiences or events in your life. It is likely that until you feel better in yourself, your weight won't change.

I find restricting any food quickly makes me feel hungry and desperate to binge on whatever it is I'm denying myself. Yes, we have to be disciplined about what we eat, and portion control is important, but a kinder approach can be trying to add in as much veg to every meal as you can. It's full of nutrients that will help you feel satisfied. If your plate is full of veg, there's not so much room for anything else. For advice on healthy eating, check out the work of Professor Tim Spector. I like his approach of trying to eat as many different plants over the course of a week as possible, and he explains more about the pernicious lobbying of the food industry to steer us all into buying highly processed foods, which ultimately can damage our health.

It's clear that for many of us, there is a lot going on behind the 'diet' side of diet and exercise. It's not as simple as telling people to eat less. With this book, my core message is to help you focus more on what your body can do and how it strong and capable it can feel. When you start to view yourself as someone who is strong and fit, you will actually *want* to make healthier food choices. If your aim is to get better at running or swimming or dancing, for example, you need to fuel your body with nutritious food to give it decent sources of energy. This will allow it to do what it needs to do in building muscle and working at its best.

Loving your body

It's not your fault if you feel bad about how you look. Social media platforms such as Instagram know full well the effect they have on people's mental health, especially on teenagers, and the amount of tweaking, photoshopping, and full-on faking that goes on in the photos of 'influencers' is downright scandalous. No one looks in real life how they look on Instagram. And yet we can't help but compare how we look to the people who seem most glamorous and successful.

Film stars go to enormous lengths so that they look like superheroes on screen. Male actors do huge amounts of muscle building and then dehydrate themselves almost to the point of collapse for one shirtless scene. They do also have a team of people to help them and their entire professional reputation depends upon it. It's not normal and not behaviour that ordinary people could or should emulate. I always find it surprising to watch TV programmes or films from the nineties and earlier—heartthrob actors look so much more NORMAL than they do now. More and more people, especially young women, are altering their bodies in real life to make themselves look more like the fake bodies they see on screen. Enormous plumped up lips, bums and boobs, and liposuctioned tummies and thighs. Botoxed foreheads, tattooed on makeup, and permanent pouts are all over any reality TV show which is aimed particularly at women and teenage girls. No matter how little attention you might think you pay to the figures you see on the screen, it seeps in.

Of course, people have always gone to great lengths to fit in with the fashions of the day. Corset, anyone? Powdered wig? Those teeny-tiny Chinese shoes? I don't suppose it has ever been easy for people to feel like they look 'right', and we humans are particularly keen on modifying our bodies and decorating them to look a certain way. It's nothing new, and the pressure doesn't seem to be going away. Remember, it's all a fashion. I am particularly relieved that I didn't over-pluck my eyebrows during the nineties when that was all the rage, so I didn't have to draw them on when thicker brows became cool again. My particular body shape hasn't been on trend for centuries, but when it comes back, I'll be ready.

Body Positivity

As a backlash to the obvious harm from social media and all this fakery, there is the body positivity, or 'health at every size' movement. Great, you might think. Let's show what 'real women' look like. Except often these 'real women' are also posing in bikinis, and it seems to polarise us even more, with people either being on the side of 'thinspirational' barbie-doll looks (because they don't want to encourage the fatties) or the 'let it all hang out and be very overweight' side. There's still not a lot of representation of slightly overweight, average looking people. Or older people. Or men of any shape and size other than tall and muscular. Many ethnic groups or people with disabilities are barely spotted in the mainstream at all. There are plenty of people still under-represented. And again, because we live in a society obsessed by visual images, it is all very much focused on what your body looks like.

I find this business of 'loving your body' a bit weird. Why should we focus on the bag of bones, flesh, and skin we find ourselves in? After all, your body pretty much does what you tell it, but should you *love* it? What happens when your body gets sick or injured? Do you still celebrate it? This self-love movement is mainly aimed at women, but what about men—should they be loving their stretch marks and wobbly bits too? Are their bodies 'amazing' whatever shape they are in?

Do you love your left elbow? The hair in your nostrils? What about all the useful mucus your body produces? Maybe I should set up an Instagram account celebrating mine. *#loveyourmucus.*

I get it that the culture of 'love your body' is trying to make people feel better about something that deep down, they don't like. A flabby, 'imperfect' body doesn't fit into society's collective view of what makes a person beautiful. However, I don't believe that this should pressure us into 'flaunting our curves', to use Daily-Mail-speak. There used to be an irritating advert on the telly where two women fling off their sarongs and march triumphantly into the sea in their bikinis like they have won some kind of battle for womankind. What do they want, a medal? Wear a bikini if you want to wear a bikini, but if you are more comfortable covered up, that's fine too.

My view is that we shouldn't be focusing on our body's appearance at all. Why spend any time trying to convince yourself that you love your body if you don't? Do you actually *need* to love how your body looks? What will you gain from it? Whatever shape you are in now, in 20 years when you look back on this time in your life, what are you going to remember? Are you going to remember what size jeans you could fit into, or would you rather remember the things you did and the fun times you had? Do you want to remember how your body looked or what you did with it?

The more attention you focus on your outward appearance, the more miserable you stand to get as you get older. Because, if things go according to plan, then you are going to get old and look old. Basing your self-esteem on how you look is not a good long-term strategy.

I have always thought that I am fat, and have spent many hours telling myself this, feeling miserable when I catch my reflection walking past a shop window, or in an unflattering photo. I have also spent a considerable amount of time creating diet plans, which I inevitably fail at after a couple of days. The phrase, "I wish I was as fat as the first time I thought I was fat," is applicable here. There were many things I didn't do and many clothes I wouldn't wear because of feeling 'too fat'. All the 'Before' pictures I've taken at the start of a diet plan could be put together to make an album showing me in my bra and knickers getting slightly fatter and older over the years.

Looking back, of course I wish I had just done the stuff I wanted to do, or worn the clothes I wanted to wear, or not wear. I certainly don't want to look back on my kids' childhood and regret that I didn't play in the pool with them, or run about in the park with them, or do fun stuff because I was worried about how flabby I might look to other people. It will not be long before my kids are teenagers and think I am the saddest, most embarrassing excuse for a human being anyway. Who wants to waste this time fretting about a bit of fat?

Perhaps we ought to all get rid of our weighing scales, mirrors and cameras for a bit. It would be quite refreshing to have no idea what I look like or how much I weigh. To live fully in the moment, like a child. I absolutely loved the fact that when they were little, my kids were completely unselfconscious about their bodies. They had strong opinions about what they wore, but it had absolutely nothing to do with how the clothes made their body look, instead it was because they wanted to be a unicorn or a ninja. My eight-year-old daughter still spends much of her time dressed as a fox.

In truth, for people outside of the evil eye of the tabloid press, nobody else really gives a monkey's about whether you are fat or thin, unless it's extreme either way and harming your health. Probably the only person telling you that you look awful... is you. Would you put up with anyone in your life speaking to you the way you speak to yourself? If you want to change your diet, go ahead, but think about it as a long-term strategy. Yes, you might be desperate for a quick fix, but short-term diets will lead to short-term results. If you want to lose some weight and keep it off for the long term, you've got to find a way of eating you can sustain and back it up with exercise and supporting your mental health.

It's not your fault if you struggle with your weight. Have a bit of compassion for yourself. You're fighting against the environment in which you live, and the body you inhabit. Don't be hard on yourself for being heavier than you want to be. The world is stacked against you being happy with your body. Think about adding good stuff in, rather than depriving yourself of anything, and get the movement bit sorted. Moving more has a knock-on positive effect as you will burn off some calories, but on a deeper level, the feeling of strength and ability that you gain from getting fitter helps your self-esteem no end, which will help you feel better about yourself. Happier people make healthier choices because they like themselves more. If you want to keep your body as the well-oiled athletic machine it can be, you'll want to nourish it with decent food, instead of drowning your negative feelings in sugar. But if and when you reach for the tub of ice cream, don't beat yourself up about it.

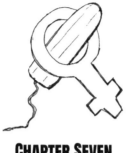

CHAPTER SEVEN

MAN, I FEEL LIKE A WOMAN

Do you have a menstrual cycle? If so, do you track it?

For those of us who have a menstrual cycle and the accompanying variation of hormones across the month (or however long your cycle is), it's well worth keeping track of what's going on with your mood, energy levels, and food cravings for a few months. Part of what is holding you back from feeling like moving could relate to a variety of what people euphemistically call 'women's issues'.

We have three main hormones in play across the month: oestrogen, progesterone and testosterone, and the way their levels change affects how you feel.

Everyone is different and some people have much more dramatic effects, while others barely notice anything.

A standard cycle goes something like this:

At the beginning of your cycle, from day 1 of your period onwards, levels of oestrogen rise. As oestrogen and testosterone levels rise, your spatial skills improve, and your social intelligence too. You should start to feel more energetic, optimistic and motivated. This might be a good time to start something new, like a new project or fitness programme. This is also a good time to focus on strength training. You may feel most anxious during this time.

Around the middle of your cycle, or 14 days before your period is due, this is when ovulation should occur. Around this time is when you could feel your most sexy.

As you head from ovulation towards your period, your oestrogen levels start to deplete, which can leave you feeling low or irritable. You might be tired or feeling weaker. You might also feel calmer than in the previous couple of weeks. Rising levels of progesterone can affect your gut, causing bloating or a change to your bowel movements. Gentler exercise, like walking or restorative yoga, might feel more palatable. During this time, I find I drop things on the floor a lot. The closer you get to your period, the less you might feel like taking on anything new, or doing anything other than curling up on the sofa with a bar of chocolate. However, the mood-boosting benefits of getting your body moving will probably help to ease feeling low or irritable at different times of your cycle. The exercise or movement you feel up to doing might change across the month, and become more gentle as the cycle progresses, so listen to your body and move accordingly.

When I'm pre-menstrual, I am useless at rock climbing, which I do every week at our local indoor climbing centre. Not only do my muscles feel weaker, but I also feel more fearful, which is a double whammy of crap when needing a load of strength to do a scary thing. But because I'm aware of the time of the month and why it's happening, I don't get upset because my abilities have suddenly plummeted (not a good word to use in relation to climbing...). Instead, on those days, I focus more on just doing easier stuff to maintain my fitness.

Why is this important?

It's important to know yourself and your own body, to know what to expect and when, and to be alert to any changes. If you struggle with a low mood in the week before your period, this might not be the best time to try to complete any new challenges or to go for your personal best in something.

It is also important to know that severely painful periods or horrendous mood swings don't have to be put up with. Just because it is normal for you or for the women in your family doesn't mean there isn't a solution. It's a slow process trying to get help for 'women's issues', and it can take a long time to get taken seriously. For example, endometriosis takes on average seven years to get diagnosed in the UK. Endometriosis causes severe, debilitating pain, so that's years and years of suffering before a diagnosis is made. If you are trying to get to the bottom of an issue, please don't give up!

There are a mix of things you can try to help even out your mood and physical symptoms over the course of your cycle. Obviously, there is the medical route. Don't listen to any women's health 'expert' who dismisses pharmaceuticals like the contraceptive pill or HRT. These are absolute life savers for many people. You can also look at your sleep, diet, exercise, stress levels and external pollutants such as chemicals in food and products we use on our skin. It's worth looking at both medical and non-medical options.

Perimenopause and Menopause

Things can go haywire during perimenopause - the years leading up to the menopause. As we get older, our oestrogen levels decline, which can cause symptoms across the whole body, affecting quality of life. Oestrogen is a hormone found in every cell, and so its decline doesn't just cause a loss of fertility. It can lead to headaches, weight gain, memory problems, anxiety, bladder weakness, sleep issues. The effects can be so serious that women end up taking themselves out of the workplace, or their relationships break down.

The drop in progesterone and testosterone also affects mental clarity, calmness and libido.

> "The low mood that can be triggered by hormonal changes is not the same as clinical depression in the typical sense. Research has shown that more than half of all perimenopausal women report an increase in depressive symptoms, but it also shows that there are differences in the nature of the low mood faced by people in the peri/menopause. The depth of sadness might not be as low as those with depression unrelated to menopause, but there can be more irritability and anger, more unwanted thoughts of worthlessness and being worried about what others think of you, a more frequent feeling of guilt, and more intrusive thoughts that may even involve suicide."[26]

If you are feeling terrible, there are a few resources out there that can help, even if your own doctor isn't very clued up on it. A good place to start is the **balance menopause** app and website.

Although you might not feel like it, you might find that doing more exercise helps with symptoms of PMS or perimenopause. Changing something else could have a bigger effect, but you won't know until you do some experimentation over the course of a few months. There are so many factors involved, it's difficult to tell what helps and what doesn't. I would suggest that exercise is definitely something to consider, especially when it can have knock-on effects on other factors. For example, if doing more exercise also helps improve your sleep and reduces stress levels, then by doing more exercise you are potentially making beneficial changes in more than one area.

It is shocking that something that half the population goes through is only recently getting attention in the public eye. Girls and boys aren't taught much about the menstrual cycle other than about periods and how not to get pregnant. We're not told what the different hormones do and how they can affect our lives. We're not told much about the menopause either, other than to expect hot flushes.

A woman is not an anomalous version of a man, and male is not the ideal that women don't live up to. We are half the population and should be treated as such. If we are expected to perform like men in the workplace throughout our lives, and keep our bodies healthy, and look after our mental health, then we need to know what is going on behind the scenes, so to speak. Otherwise, how can we know the signs to look out for and when we should ask for help?

The Pelvic Floor

While we're discussing things that affect women, something that affects a lot of women is weakness in the pelvic floor. Again, this is another huge topic that has been massively overlooked by mainstream health and fitness professionals, to the point that adverts for incontinence pads are regularly seen on the TV and it seems to be a bigger industry teaching people how to put up with the problem rather than how to prevent or repair it.

What 'treatments' there are have turned out to make matters irrevocably worse for some: there has been a recent scandal in the UK about incorrectly fitted vaginal mesh implants that have caused many hundreds of women permanent life-changing damage.

When we talk about the pelvic floor, we are talking about a hammock of muscles that sits across the base of the pelvis, between the pubic bone and tail bone and from side to side. These muscles support the bladder, bowel and the uterus, as well as stabilising your spine, controlling the pressure in your abdomen, and playing an important role in sex: both in sensation and function.

Pelvic floor weakness can affect anyone, male or female, but it is most commonly seen in women who have had a baby and older women. A weak pelvic floor can lead to stress incontinence (letting out a bit of wee when laughing, or running, for example), erectile dysfunction in men, and pelvic organ prolapse. Maybe when you need the toilet, you need to go - now.

Pelvic floor issues can result from the muscles being too weak or too tight. We often assume that if we have a problem with a muscle it's because it is too weak and we need to strengthen it. This may be the case, but it could also be the case that you've been holding it tight for too long and you have lost the ability to relax it.

The standard exercise for the pelvic floor is the 'Kegel', which is where you squeeze and hold the muscles, like when stopping the flow of urine, and then relax. You can find loads of advice on how to do this and even apps and devices to help you train your pelvic floor.

Kegels are only part of the story, and it is worth looking into this deeper. Once again, I recommend Katy Bowman's work, as she makes the excellent point that as the pelvic floor muscles are connected to other muscles, we need to look at how all these muscles align and work with one another. Kegels on their own probably won't suffice. This is a long quote from an excellent blog post that I highly recommend you read:

> "I do get the need for therapeutic/corrective exercise (I teach many of these exercises and I think they are great), and I even see a place for Kegel exercises as a beginning step to moving pelvis-parts more. But my main point in the great Kegel debates is this:

a single exercise to competently train an area of the body with so much depending upon it won't cut it, and thinking that one small exercise will suffice is the approach a sedentary culture will keep trying to take, an approach that will keep getting poor results. **We must talk about this giant sedentary vacuum, sucking out all the movement from our lives.** If we can't get our culture moving, human movement will be reduced to a list of therapeutic exercises to be done to improve a part/symptom (a part suffering or symptom arising often from a lack of movement), from here on out. We won't see movement as part of the medicine wheel of our lives. We won't understand that movement—whole-body, whole-life movement—is as essential to our health and vitality as water or air."[27]

The article can be found on Katy's Nutritious Movement website at: nutritiousmovement.com/my-pelvic-position-in-2020. In addition, if you have problems with your pelvic floor function, look for a specialist near you who can help.

Being sedentary doesn't help pelvic floor function, perimenopausal symptoms or the ability to cope with hormonal variation across the menstrual cycle. Moving more of your body more often is a potential solution to all of these issues and once again highlights how being sufficiently active is not just about looking good. It is vital to every body in almost every way.

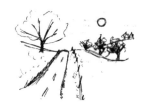

CHAPTER EIGHT

LET'S GO OUTSIDE

Exercise and movement are important, but we try to avoid it wherever possible, with good reason. How can we find ways to *want* to exercise and keep on wanting to exercise? What should we do when we don't feel motivated? How can we make movement a part of life, and what has been holding us back from this before now?

Light and Space

Want more energy? Go outside. It's natural to want to move more out in the fresh air than when you're cooped up inside with all the various sedentary distractions.

Living in the UK, the climate means going outside is not always a very appealing proposition. But even in the dreariest weather there are benefits to be gained.

We all have a circadian rhythm, which is the hard-wired, 24-hour body clock in our brains which tells us when we should be awake and when we should be asleep. The trouble is that modern life can screw up this rhythm by giving us too much light when we should be getting sleepy, and not enough light when we should be waking up.

Ideally, we need lots of bright daylight as soon as possible after waking up and we should avoid light when it's time to prepare for sleep. However, if we spend our evenings with loads of bright screens, the blue light from these hits your brain and inhibits the correct function of the body clock, meaning that it can be much more difficult to fall asleep. We know how important decent sleep is, and if you want to move more and exercise more, you're going to need energy and you're going to need to get enough sleep. Assuming you're not a night-shift worker, or don't have a non-sleeping child to look after, it's well worth trying to prioritise things that will help you sleep.

In the Northern Hemisphere winter, many of us never get outside to see any daylight at all, when it is dark before and after work. But if it's at all possible to get outside during the morning, even just for a ten-minute coffee break, then it's worth doing. If you are choosing to do some exercise outside, going out first thing in the morning will give you a double whammy of benefits.

Why else is getting outside so important?

Going outside is not just about getting your body clock functioning properly. It is also useful for relaxation, for stimulating your senses, and for reducing anxiety. By researching Japanese 'forest bathing', we can discover why this is:

Forest bathing

Forest bathing involves going and spending time among trees or other natural places, being slow, calm and quiet, breathing deeply and taking in your surroundings. It seems obvious that being in a calm, natural environment will leave you feeling more relaxed, but why?

Being in nature can help to lower blood pressure, reduce levels of the stress hormone, cortisol, and even support your immune system's 'natural killer' cells, which fight cancer, infections and inflammation. It turns out that trees give off essential oils containing chemicals called phytoncides, and studies in Japan have shown that exposure to phytoncides may contribute to increased activity of these beneficial natural killer cells.[28]

You don't have to hug a tree for hours to get the benefits. Half an hour a week will help:

> "A dose-response analysis for depression and high blood pressure suggest that visits to outdoor green spaces of 30 minutes or more during the course of a week could reduce the population prevalence of these illnesses by up to 7% and 9% respectively."[29]

Forest bathing is straightforward. Use all your senses: Notice not just the sights, but the sounds, smells, and feel of the area you are in. If you're wondering about the sense of taste, maybe don't go licking the trees (not when anyone's watching, at least), but instead notice the taste of the air and how fresh it is compared with indoors. Using all your senses in this way is a very meditative practice and allows you to be fully in the moment. It might be difficult at first, but just trying it will be good for you.

If you don't have a nearby forest, you can get the same effect from any natural landscape, even a city park if you can find a quiet spot.

Outside is interesting

Moving and exercising outside is usually more interesting than indoors, meaning you'll want to keep going for longer. Using a treadmill or riding an exercise bike is considerably more boring than going outside for the same activity. I suppose you can watch the TV or listen to music while exercising indoors, but it's also a lot easier to stop when you're on an indoor machine than when you've already got yourself a mile or so away from home.

Outside there is more to look at and your brain needs to be more engaged to avoid obstacles or not get lost, which makes the time go faster. You can spot signs of the changing seasons, helping you feel more connected to your environment and the natural world around you. You can find beauty in even the smallest patches of nature, like the way tiny, fragile weeds push through the cracks in the pavement or grow up a wall. We love to look at interesting landscapes, whether urban, beach, or rural. After all, a room with a view is rather more desirable than a cell with no window.

Grounding

It can also be really calming to feel the solid earth beneath your feet. We can get caught up with what's going on in our heads and the breath moves up into the throat. All the tension seems to rise up, up, up. By focusing down into the ground and feeling the soles of your feet connecting to the earth, it can bring the tension and anxiety down. As you breathe, imagine roots coming out of the bottom of your feet, connecting you to the earth.

Try Camping!

It's a bit of a love-it-or-hate-it activity, but in my experience, going camping really supports the idea that we should spend more time outside. On paper, everything about camping is hard work, uncomfortable and tiring. The toilet facilities, for a start, are not of a standard I usually demand. Preparing food or hot drinks is a lot more time-consuming, there's no dishwasher, and worst of all, there's no comfy bed.

However, illogical as it might seem, I love camping. We have spent a few years building up the right kit, which helps. Even though I don't sleep terribly well, I feel refreshed and relaxed, and I'm convinced it's because of being outside all the time. I get natural daylight all day, and also much more movement as every task is a lot less convenient than at home. Most of the equipment is at ground level, requiring lots of squatting or bending down and lifting things. It's usually a fair walk to the nearest tap, so water has to be carried. Camping chairs are less easy to lounge on, and the kids spend a huge amount of time running around, playing with new friends, which they would never do at home. There is very little screen time and a lot more gazing into the distance. It's all time spent around greenery too. I can't deny it's good to get home to my own shower, and it's utterly miserable in the rain, but I dream of sitting by the campfire, drinking wine out of a tin mug.

When you live in a town like I do, it's very easy to fall into the habit of being a very indoor creature. One thing the Covid-19 pandemic has shown us is that when being outside is the only option for socialising or exercising, it is possible and even enjoyable. We don't always have to sit inside in the pub or exercise indoors in a gym. We can have coffee with a friend in the park instead of inside a café.

If something can be done outdoors, choose that option. The weather isn't always kind to us, and most of us don't live somewhere stunning with panoramic views, but it doesn't always rain all day, and wherever we are we can usually find a view that we find pleasant or interesting—or just stand outside your door and look up.

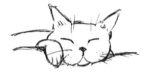

CHAPTER NINE

GETTING MORE REST

Taking a break

You don't need me to tell you that life is stressful. Exercise is helpful for dealing with stress, but so is learning how to rest. You might think you don't need to learn how to rest, but just lounging around isn't really resting. Just because you are physically still doesn't mean that you are actually relaxing, or that your mind is allowing your body to stop producing stress hormones.

It can help just to be aware throughout your day whether or not you are tense. If you work at a desk, notice what happens when you open your emails or start typing something. Are your shoulders tense? Have you stopped breathing? I have a tendency to hold my breath when I'm working, and I don't realise I'm doing it. Stopping every so often to roll my shoulders and readjust my posture helps prevent shoulder and neck pain, and focusing on breathing makes my body relax. After all, I don't need tense muscles to type an email, but I end up creating tension in my system and producing stress hormones when they really aren't needed. Check in with yourself throughout the day and see how relaxed or tense you are. Are you clenching your teeth or frowning? You can trick your body into calming down just by acting as a calm body would. Fake it until you make it really works.

A great big sigh

When you notice you are uptight or stressed, there's an effective technique to calm your system instantly, called a "physiological sigh". Here's how you do it: take one deep breath in, through your nose, until your lungs feel full; then immediately take another breath in, like a big sniff—quickly this time. Now, breathe out slowly. This second breath in gets the alveoli (air sacs) in your lungs to pop open, allowing twice the volume of a normal breath. This means more oxygen goes in, and also more carbon dioxide goes out. If something bad happens, we hold our breath or start breathing more shallowly, which means carbon dioxide builds up in the bloodstream. An increased volume of carbon dioxide in your blood triggers the release of stress hormones, because it's telling your body there's a problem. An enormous sigh which gets lots of oxygen in and lots of carbon dioxide out is saying that the stress response isn't necessary and you calm down.

Other ways to chill out

Getting outside whenever you can is also really calming, for all the reasons mentioned in the previous chapter. I used to teach parenting classes to parents of newborn babies, and one of the best pieces of advice when you've got a crying baby is to take them outside. It's amazing how often the baby will stop crying as soon as they are out in the fresh air. I'm not sure how much of that is because the fresh air calms the baby, and how much is because the fresh air calms the parent, which calms the baby. Either way, getting outside is calming. Going back to the evolution thing, early humans would have spent a lot of time outside. If you can see what's going on around you, you know you are safe when you can see there are no threats approaching.

A second piece of advice I used to give parents of colicky babies, i.e., babies who had long periods of inconsolable, unexplained crying, was to get them in the bath. The only thing that would calm my daughter as a newborn was to get in the bath with her. She would lie on my chest with the warm water lapping around her and she would miraculously stop crying. A warm bath relaxes most of us. We spent the most stress-free months of our lives in the womb surrounded by warm water, so it makes sense that it is a pleasant feeling.

The third and final thing that works best of all for babies and adults is to be held. Babies just want to be held. If they are crying, pick them up. It reduces their stress levels to be held in loving arms. Skin to skin contact is incredibly calming, and premature babies are given 'kangaroo care', where they are held against an adult's chest, skin to skin, and wrapped up in a special t-shirt or sling to hold them there nice and tight.

Having a hug with someone you trust will have a relaxing effect on you, too. A 20-second hug seems quite long, but that's how long it can take for you to relax into it. Human contact and touch are vital to our wellbeing, so go and find someone to hug.

In looking at how we can make our bodies fitter and readier for taking on the world, I don't think we can leave out training your brain from the equation. After all, it's no good to just get your body in good shape, if your mind is a mess, which brings us to looking at how to relax - mentally.

Proper Relaxation

Deep relaxation, mindfulness, meditation, call it what you will, learning how to do it can teach your brain new and improved ways to deal with stress and anxiety.

There are many different types of meditation and it has been around for thousands of years, so while terms like 'mindfulness meditation' may seem like a new trend, the core practice is ancient. It's definitely worth taking some techniques from meditation practices to switch off the nagging, stressing, repetitive voice in our heads that keeps us in a state of anxiety or worry, and allow us to have just a few moments of calm. When you learn how to feel completely relaxed, it's a state you can get yourself back into more easily each time you need to.

You may think you can't alter your own mental state without drugs or alcohol, but we do actually go in and out of different states all day long. Have you ever been driving along and suddenly realised you have no recollection of how you got to where you are now? You must have been driving safely because there's no trail of destruction in your wake, but your mind was elsewhere and something automatic had taken over to keep you on the road.

Have you ever got so absorbed in an activity that you completely lost track of time? This is called a state of flow. Flow is something to pursue as much as possible. If you find something that you really love to do and that completely absorbs your attention, then make it a priority to do it. It's great for your brain. This could be playing a video game, doing puzzles, playing music, swimming, knitting, painting.

It is possible to learn how to relax. We all have the tools at our disposal, but if you have been stressed out for a while, you've probably not been properly relaxed for some time. You're aiming to feel soft and loose throughout your entire body, not holding onto any tension anywhere.

Focusing on your breathing is useful because there is a feedback loop between your brain and your breath. If you breathe like a relaxed person, your brain thinks there is nothing to worry about and will send the message to your body that you are safe and you can be calm. If you breathe like there's a scary monster just around the corner, i.e., fast, shallow breaths, the message goes back to your brain that it's time to get the hell out of there. Your body will become flooded with stress hormones and your muscles will tense up in readiness for fight or flight. Breathe like this all the time and your brain thinks you're always in danger.

How to breathe

Yes, you know how to breathe. But do you know how to calm yourself through your breath? To teach yourself to breathe calmly, all you need to do is focus on slow, gentle breaths. The out-breath needs to be longer than the in-breath. Counting can help, so you can breathe in for a count of four and out for a count of six. You can do what's known as 3, 4, 5 breathing, where you breathe in for a count of 3, hold your breath for a count of 4, and breathe out for a count of 5. There is also 'box breathing' where you imagine you are breathing around the sides of a box, so you breathe in as you imagine travelling along one side of the box, hold your breath for the second side, exhale for the third side and hold for the fourth side. It doesn't really matter how you do it, as long as you breathe slowly and steadily and keep the exhale nice and long.

If you're doing one of these breathing exercises and focusing on your breath, maybe counting as you do it, then congratulations, you're meditating. Get yourself in a comfortable position and try doing this breathing for just two minutes. See how you feel afterwards. Once you have got the hang of doing two minutes of nice relaxing breathing, you might feel like trying a body scan practice. This one is my favourite for helping me get to sleep, and it works really well for children too.

Body scan relaxation practice

To help your body fully relax, lie in a comfortable position on your back on the floor or a bed, and make sure you're warm enough. Begin by tensing the muscles in your toes and hold them tight for a second or two, then relax and allow them to go completely soft and floppy. Really think about your toes. Try to get your mind to focus fully on them so that you are very aware of them. Where are they in space? How do they feel? Can you bring your awareness to each toe?

Next, do the same for the soles of your feet, your heels, your ankles, and gradually work your way up every bit of your body, down your arms, and even your face and scalp. Take your time to focus on each body part, making sure nowhere gets missed out. Tense and relax each part before you move up to the next part.

When you have done this, your whole body should be completely relaxed. It should feel like you almost can't move your arms and legs, as they have become so limp. Take a few moments to enjoy this sensation of relaxation. It is important to notice how you are feeling at this moment. You might feel very sleepy. Can you notice the difference between how you feel now and how you felt when you started? I hold a lot of tension in my throat and upper chest, so I make a point of noticing when that area relaxes and how nice it feels. You might hold tension somewhere else. Is your jaw relaxed? Are your shoulders down from up near your ears? Is your forehead smooth or frowning? Have you unclenched your fists? By focusing on each part of your body in turn, not only does it allow you to fully relax your muscles and leave no part still tensed up, but it also means that the entire time you are doing this exercise, your mind is engaged in focusing on your body, and not any of the things that you have been worrying about until now. When you find your mind wandering, just gently go back to the part of the body you have got up to. It's not a problem if you can't do the whole thing in one go, or if you think about other things, that's completely normal and to be expected. Every minute you spend doing this is a minute well spent.

It's good for your digestion too. You might notice that your stomach gurgles as you get more relaxed. This is a good sign, as it shows that your body can finally digest your food. When you are in a state of high alert, the blood flow diverts to the muscles in the arms and legs, so you're primed and ready to deal with the threat. But this means that the focus is not on digestion, which can lead to unpleasant side effects. However, when you are nice and relaxed, the blood can go back to the organs and get on with things like digesting food properly.

If you like how this practice makes you feel, stick with it, or investigate other ways to meditate or be mindful. You can use it to switch off worries in the present moment, to help you sleep, to start your day on a calm and focused note, or to promote feelings of love and kindness towards others. A few moments of changing your focus can help before doing a task you're nervous about, and it can help when dealing with troublesome people, too. It's a skill you will have to put some effort into learning, but you don't need to go on ten-day silent retreats to get the benefits—just a couple of minutes at a time can be helpful enough.

Will all this change my life?

Learning to relax won't deal with the root cause of whatever is stressing you out. Getting fitter and all the benefits that brings also won't solve your problems. However, they are useful tools and there's nothing wrong with using them as a sticking plaster. Making relaxation a priority will have physical benefits. It can give you relief and teach you new coping mechanisms. Learning how to cope with uncomfortable feelings and managing stress is useful in all areas of life, including in making changes and leaving our comfort zone when it comes to exercise and fitness. Being able to relax and escape the stressed-out fight-or-flight state will also allow your body to rest and recover, helping your muscles, digestion, and stress hormone levels. Being calmer will give you the mental clarity to see where you can make changes and feeling more rested will give you more energy when you need it.

For some people, getting into exercise or meditation comes at the right moment and does absolutely change their life, but don't trust anyone who promises it's going to be a panacea for all your ills. The 'wellness' space has a tendency to promise people that if you eat like this, practice this form of exercise, or this self-care routine, you'll be as fit and slim and carefree as the person promoting it. This probably doesn't come from a disingenuous place, as it's understandable that when someone finds something that works for them, they want to tell the world and help as many people as possible. Just be wary if it seems too good to be true.

Notice if you are physically tense or stressed. Do you need to be? Are you in imminent physical danger? Calm yourself down with a breathing exercise, get outside or hug someone. If you've got more time, have a warm bath or do some relaxing meditation—either the body scan described here or listen to a guided one.

The Wheel of Life

While we're looking at being calmer and feeling better about things, if you are interested in how to be healthy and happy, you need to look at your life as a whole. You can be the fittest person in the world, but still feel like crap because your marriage is breaking down, for instance. You might find that there's an area of your life that you hadn't really considered, which is making you feel low overall. I like to use an exercise I learned in some performance coaching training, which lays it out in a nice, visual way:

Draw a circle and split it into eight sections so it looks like a wheel. Each spoke on the wheel represents an area of your life which affects your health and wellbeing. You can choose your own areas, but these usually cover it:

1. Food/diet

2. Movement/fitness

3. Health

4. Friends/family

5. Spirituality/living in accordance with your values

6. Intimate relationship

7. Work/career

8. Finances

You might like to include one for other areas like living arrangements or material possessions. You might find you need to split friends and family into two separate segments. 'Sleep' might be another category to add, if that's something you struggle with or don't get enough of. The categories mean whatever they mean to you—only you know what's most important to you in your life.

Number 5 doesn't have to be about religion, unless you are religious. Even if you are completely atheist, it's still important for all of us to live a life that we feel is in line with our values and beliefs, whatever a 'good life' means to you. This can be completely secular, like acts of kindness, good deeds for others, or even spending enough time on your own self-care. Humans benefit from being in communion with something that is bigger than ourselves, feeling part of a bigger picture, and that's what this area relates to.

When you have drawn your wheel, you'll end up with something that looks like this:

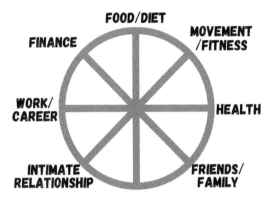

The next stage is to give a score for each area. The centre of the wheel is zero out of ten - the worst it could possibly be, and the outer edge of the wheel is ten out of ten - the best it could possibly be. Now, you can score each area out of ten. So, my scores might be:

1. Food/diet = 7

2. Movement/fitness = 8

3. Health = 9

4. Friends/family = 7

5. Spirituality/living in accordance with values = 10

6. Intimate relationship = 8

7. Work/career = 5

8. Finance = 5

Next, I can roughly plot these numbers on my wheel:

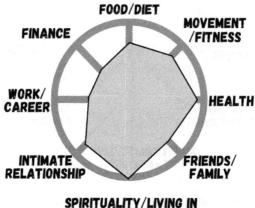

The bigger your shape, the happier you are with your life overall. If, for example, I had just lost my job and scored Work/Career as a 1 or a zero, you can see what effect that would have on the shape of my wheel. It wouldn't work terribly well on a bicycle. Similarly, when I had young children who woke me up every two hours for the first couple of years of their lives, no matter how good any other aspects of my life were, my wheel would still be wonky. I was exhausted all the time, and so that had a knock-on effect on all the other areas, making my wheel look like one on a clown's tiny bicycle.

Like any personality test, the Wheel of Life only tells you something about how you are feeling at the moment you fill it in. It's a useful exercise to see how you feel about your life overall and which areas you feel are going better than others. I like it because it gives me clarity on why I might feel down or lethargic. The reason I've included it here is as a reminder that while fitness might be one area of your life you're not happy with, if there are other things going on don't expect miracles from sorting out just one area.

Filling in the wheel might also show you why feeling stuck or unhappy with your fitness level isn't something you should be cross with yourself about: yes, your fitness might be poor, but that's because your toddler wakes you up three times a night, or because you have an insanely busy job, or because you have absolutely no time to yourself because of caring responsibilities. Everything is related; it is all part of the same wheel.

It's also worth remembering that we shouldn't ever expect to be ten out of ten in all areas. There are always going to be setbacks and difficulties in life.

If there are fundamental things in your life that need to be changed before you can be truly content, no amount of running or meditating is going to fix it. It may not be in your power to make those changes. However, making sure you look after your body by giving it the things it needs certainly won't do any harm, and is likely to give you a bit of a lift. It can help get you through difficult times when you might otherwise not have been able to hold it together, giving you new tools and coping mechanisms, and making you feel stronger and more capable.

Sometimes doing something new will give you a different perspective on life and show you how things could be different. Doing what you have always done will get you what you always got, so what have you got to lose? You might meet new people or discover new places. Or you might find just having half an hour away from your family to relax or move is enough to get you through the rest of the day without screaming at anyone.

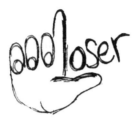

CHAPTER TEN

WHY AM I SO BAD AT THIS?

Many of us who have never been keen on exercise or sport believe it is because it's just something we are no good at. We've always been rubbish and we're too old to start now. Is this really true, or could we perhaps stop being so hard on ourselves?

Common excuse number one: I am too old to get fit.

What sort of old person do you want to be? You are still going to feel like you on the inside, no matter what the outside looks like. Do you want to be sitting in your armchair all day, grumbling at the TV and waiting for your family to come and visit? Or do you want to be buying your first motorbike, donning some leathers and going off on adventures?

If you want to have a go at something new, the best time to start is now. You're only going to get older anyway, so what's the worst that can happen? If you want to try something that takes place in a club, then check them out. See how you feel about the instructor. It might surprise you to see people even older than you there, crushing it with the young 'uns. At our local rock climbing centre I've seen people of all ages, shapes and sizes on the wall—men and women in their 60s and 70s, who climb stuff I can't. I've been to gym classes with people in their 60s and 70s too. And yoga, Pilates, swimming, Park Run, and walking groups. If you find something you love - don't stop, and if you haven't found the thing yet, there's still time.

You won't build muscle as quickly as when you were younger, and you may be less flexible and at a higher risk of injury. But that's no reason not to have a go. As we've already seen, there are massive health benefits to being active as you get older.

Humans are unusual in that we don't just die when our reproductive years are over. We evolved to be useful as grandparents as well as parents. Grandparents play an important role in the tribe, working and looking after grandchildren so the parents can work. We ought to think of our retirement years as being equally active as our younger years. This is not the time to put your feet up for good, or you'll wither away. The activities you do might change, but the advantages to your mental and physical health of staying active as you age are abundantly clear.

Common excuse number two: I have always been useless at exercise.

Imagine the scene: You are jogging along at a steady pace on a route you do every week. You always run at the same speed. That's just the speed you go. One day when you are doing your jog, every couple of minutes someone comes along and overtakes you. They breeze past you like it's nothing. After the third or fourth person overtakes you, how do you feel? A bit demoralised? Like you're a crap runner?

The next week you go out jogging again and your speed is exactly the same as before. However, this time you find you are the one doing the overtaking. You overtake one person who seems to be running really slowly, and a few hundred metres down the path, you overtake someone else. By the time you've finished your run, you've overtaken half a dozen people, and it felt easy. You didn't have to push yourself. In fact, it was a breeze. You are the definition of athleticism and speed. How different do you feel from last week's run?

But when you go home and look at your stats on your app, you see that your performance on both runs is exactly the same.

The same could apply to lifting weights, swimming, cycling, or anything where you can see other people doing the same thing at the same time. We really mess it up for ourselves by comparing ourselves with others. What matters is seeing how different today's jog was to last month's or last year's attempt.

I'm no different from anyone else in comparing myself unfavourably with others, but I remind myself that it's the effort I'm putting in that is the important thing. If I'm putting in effort, my fitness will improve—maybe not as quickly as I'd like it to, but whatever my performance looks like on the outside, the benefits are happening on the inside. And if I want to be competitive about it, I can remind myself that those people who find it so easy aren't working as hard as I am, so I win the medal for trying the hardest.

We also need to be careful who we are comparing ourselves with. I have to train twice as hard to be half as good as my husband, who seems to have a natural affinity for running, jumping and climbing. Yes, I am utterly hopeless *compared with him*, but that doesn't mean I am actually utterly hopeless. I wouldn't compare my 100-metre sprint time with Usain Bolt's. I was going to say that I wouldn't compare my marathon time with Paula Radcliffe's, but then I remembered I can't run a marathon.

They say we are the sum total of the people we spend the most time with. If you are surrounded by people who put you down or tell you that you are not good enough, maybe you need to find a different group of people to hang out with.

What is stopping me from sticking at exercising?

Now, I like excuses and use them a lot. I'm not the sort of person to shout phrases like, "No excuses!" That road leads to things like Bootcamps and blowing whistles. I'd prefer to look at what is causing the excuses in the first place, because perhaps there is something underlying your quitter tendencies. Have a think about the following questions:

- Am I worried that I will fail?

- Do I already feel like a failure, so what's the point?

- Does something about exercise trigger painful memories from the past?

- Do I dislike myself?

- Do I feel unworthy of health and happiness?

- Am I wracked with guilt and shame for taking time for myself?

These are deep questions and are worth taking some time to consider - maybe go for a walk to ponder them. If you answer 'yes' to any of the questions above, this may explain why, despite many attempts in the past, you just can't make exercising a part of your life.

Have compassion for yourself. Wherever these feelings have come from and whatever it was in your past that has led to you feeling like this today, it isn't your fault. Whatever the underlying reasons which are holding you back from fully embracing change, they are not insurmountable. Start small.

Action figures: why do some people find it so easy to exercise?

We all know people who are superb at Doing. They are amazing at getting things done. They have a new idea and before you know it, they've done it: they started the business; they ran the marathon; they are in a new relationship, however ill-advised. They don't spend weeks and weeks over-thinking and finding reasons why it's not a good idea. If their idea isn't a success, they have an excuse why and they move on. They are always on to the next big idea, the next project. And they never seem to stop. How do they have so much energy? How do they have so many ideas?

What is it that makes some people so good at action, while others procrastinate, find excuses, and think themselves out of acting on good ideas?

Getting stuff done is satisfying. Over-thinking is not. However, there is a difference between people who start projects and actually finish them, and people who start something then abandon it at the first sign of difficulty before moving onto the next fantastic shiny new idea.

With exercise, you know why you need to exercise and you probably have a pretty good idea how to do it. So why is it you are sitting here reading, rather than getting on with actually doing the thing?

We all get into habits, and over-thinking can become a habit. Have you got into a habit of not acting on your ideas? I know I have. The coronavirus lockdowns in 2020 and 2021 were especially bad for me for this reason. I became used to not being able to do anything, and both the government and society encouraged me to do precisely nothing. Sit at home, don't go out. Don't. Do. Anything. It's a scary, dangerous world out there.

It's not entirely the pandemic's fault. I've always been biased towards thinking rather than doing, but my behaviour was reinforced during that period. It's so much easier to put off something that might be risky or uncomfortable until tomorrow, or some unspecified date in the future. I have said to myself, "It's already October, so I'll start that diet in the New Year..."

This is yet another example of us humans making things harder for ourselves, despite trying to make life easier. We tell ourselves it's safer not to try something new, not to act on an idea, and we can conjure up as many reasons as we need to put ourselves off. I had better not go for a run, as runners are always injuring themselves. I had better not go out on my bike because of all the traffic on the road. And I'm certainly not going to join the gym because what if I do something wrong and people laugh at me? But if we just got on and did it, we would feel good about ourselves for having done it, as well as any physical benefits the exercise would give us.

Perhaps you need to look at what ways of thinking have been stopping you from doing what you want to do. No doubt you are busy and have a lot on, but you want to exercise, you want to move. Does the thought of committing to something new make you anxious? Are you already coming up with reasons why it won't work? Maybe you give it a go for a couple of weeks, but as soon as there's an obstacle in the way or someone makes a critical comment, you give up? What is it you are actually scared of?

The first step to making any change is awareness. Notice your patterns of thinking. Become aware of your negative thoughts. If you have had bad associations with exercise in the past, then it's even more likely that you are going to be thinking negative thoughts about exercise—maybe even the word 'exercise' makes you shudder. Don't call it 'exercise' if the word is unpleasant to you.

The thing is, thoughts are just traffic passing through your head. It can be a busy motorway in there. You don't have to stop each car and pay attention to it. You can stand back and let the traffic pass. What is the mood inside each of those little cars in your head? Has the driver got road rage? Are they calm and happy and enjoying the flow? Are they anxious or sad?

It's difficult to separate yourself from your thoughts, and it's something that Buddhist monks take a lifetime of practice to master. But you can notice what's going on in there. What *are* your thoughts? Can you try to step back from the motorway occasionally to see what is really going on? Maybe you will realise every time you think about doing some exercise, some little voice in your head pops up and gives you a reason why you shouldn't. Is it even *your* voice, or is it the voice of someone who said something mean to you in the past?

What's Your Culture?

We live in a sedentary culture here in the UK. But on a smaller scale, what is your family culture like when it comes to movement? Do you have active friends and family? When you get together, is it normal to go for a walk, or to play sports together?

Perhaps when you were little, no one around you was into exercise. I'm lucky in that I come from a very active family and for me it was normal for various family members to be busy doing different sports and activities and for them to take priority. There's very little that my dad will cancel his Sunday cricket for, and if we want Dad to be at a family get-together, we plan it around his matches. In my wider family there are dancers, tennis players, more cricketers, rugby players, horse riders, golfers, keen gardeners, walkers. Growing up, we lived in the countryside and had lots of animals that needed looking after, firewood to chop, and a dog that needed walking. There was always something active to be doing. So, for me, being active is just what you do. I don't understand the family obsession with tennis *at all*, but being around all that sportiness means that it is ingrained into my psyche that being active is part of life.

If you don't have that background and you haven't spent your formative years with anyone who has influenced you to be active, it's completely understandable that physical activity will not be on your list as a 'must do'. It is hard to do something different from your cultural norms and it'll push you out of your comfort zone.

Realising what's normal for the people closest to you will make a difference. So much of becoming more active is about noticing what's going on. The actual movement bit and fitting it in to your life will become easier when you realise what's actually happening and where you can make small tweaks. You could also take it upon yourself to ensure that your loved ones become more active too, so you might start dragging the family out for walks or encouraging your mates to join you in your active endeavours. They'll thank you for it - maybe...

I figure that every time my kids see me doing some yoga in the living room, or insisting we walk rather than drive into town, that even if they couldn't think of anything worse right now, I am a role model for them and what I do will affect what they think is normal. You can start new traditions in your family, break cycles, start afresh.

Am I just downright lazy?

Unfit people are NOT lazy. The fact is, your energy is rightly focussed elsewhere, whether that's work, caring responsibilities, or coping with your own mental or physical health. It might be invisible work, but it's still work. We each only have a certain number of resources available, whether that's physical or mental energy, or hours in the day, and it's not possible just to create more. If you're working, looking after others, looking after the house, worrying about the many things there are to worry about, you do not have the space and time available to you to consider eating healthy foods or taking exercise. Even the people who appear to be the best at getting things done have areas of their life where they have to let things slide. We all have our own priorities because we have to. There simply isn't enough time to do everything.

I have seen life coaches break down the hours in the day to say, well, you sleep for 7 hours, you go to work for 9 hours, that leaves you EIGHT WHOLE HOURS every day to spend going to the gym or generally improving yourself. Hang on a minute, no one has a spare 8 hours a day to spend on self-improvement.

There are some ridiculous magazine articles that describe the daily habits of the highly successful person. It usually goes something like: rich and famous person gets up at 5am, spends half an hour meditating, drinks something green, works out for an hour; then they shower, go to work, and the day continues. They eat very little except supplements and ingredients you've never heard of and drink a lot of weird teas. Every minute is accounted for, and most importantly, productive. This is nonsense. These people never look after anyone else. There's no laundry, no supermarket shop, no cleaning or picking up other people's pants or dirty tissues off the floor. There's no taking the bin out and finding the bin bag has leaked all over the bottom of the bin, so you clean that up and clean the floor where you put the bin bag down. Then you have to go outside in the rain, unlock the gate, go round the side of the house, drag the bin round the front, go back inside, find a new bin bag, and so on and so forth. A tiny little job can take up an inordinate amount of time. If you're not feeling your best, then just emptying the bin can actually become quite a major task.

The problem is that we have been conditioned to think that these ultra-high achievers are aspirational. We should aim to be super productive. Idleness is bad. If you haven't got goals and ambitions, then what the hell are you doing with your life? No matter how embellished the articles about the daily life of the high achievers are, a bit of that seeps into your brain. This person is slim, gorgeous and successful and I'm not. Maybe it's me that's the problem? Then you add in the messages about diet and fitness that if you aren't slim and fit, then you just aren't trying; it's no wonder we hate ourselves for being 'fat' and 'lazy'. We're constantly told it's all our fault.

In his *Pensées*, first published in 1670, the French philosopher and mathematician Blaise Pascal, wrote the much-quoted:

> "I have often said that the sole cause of man's unhappiness is that he does not know how to stay quietly in his room."

In the health and wellness arena, I see many people putting so much effort into 'optimising' their lives. Tweaking what and when they eat to the point where their diets become extremely restrictive and pretty strange. I mean, how has it become a thing to whisk butter and coconut oil into your coffee? Wellness enthusiasts plan their exercise routines to have their heart rate at a certain level for a set amount of time; they monitor their sleep with devices. I can tell you whether I've had enough sleep without a machine to track it. Why this quest for perfection? Where's the freedom and joy? What does spending so much time and effort on self-improvement really achieve? I interpret the Pascal quote to mean that we should be able to sit with ourselves as we are now. Why are we running away from ourselves all the time?

Of course, nowadays there is an added problem that when we're sitting alone in our rooms, we're not really alone when there's a phone in our hands. So much of our social life can be completely sedentary for kids and adults alike. We can conduct life through a screen, whether that's gaming with friends or keeping up with social media. My son doesn't have to walk to the park to hang out with his mates, he just turns on the computer and there they all are. Again, it's not laziness, it's what passes for a normal life nowadays.

The more miserable you are, the less you want to move and enjoy your body. You just want to curl up in a ball—you don't want to go out and kick one about. Social media and the news make us miserable, and it's easy to see how we get into downward spirals. We don't feel like going out and moving or attempting to make something healthy to eat, all we have the energy for is lying on the sofa mindlessly doom-scrolling our phones, which only make us feel worse as we're shown people arguing with one another and telling us we're all going to die, or irritatingly frolicking about 'living their best life'. Unfortunately, we are attracted to misery. It's a survival mechanism from the most ancient parts of our brains. If you know what the dangers are and you feel fearful, in theory it will help to keep you safe, but it's not a recipe for energy and vitality, is it?

Chilling out is a good thing. We all need to rest and relax. We need time to think and to contemplate, time to reconnect with friends and family, and just enjoy life. It's essential for body and mind. It's also essential for body and mind to incorporate movement into our days, but we can do this in a quiet and gentle way. Perhaps you could walk to a friend's house or the pub, or potter in the garden. You could get an arm workout by kneading some bread dough. Perhaps download an audiobook to listen to while you walk or do jobs around the house. Try some yoga stretches and meditation in your living room. It involves changing your mindset to become happier with a life where you compare yourself less with others and say a mental 'sod off' to anyone implying that because you don't look like a beautiful, over-achieving, celebrity that you are at fault.

Just because you aren't spending every minute of every day in a productive whirl, optimising all areas of your life and running marathons doesn't mean you are lazy and doesn't mean you are bad. You can choose to reframe being imperfect as a positive, radical act of fighting against a system that makes money from your dissatisfaction. You can also find ways to move your body that will help you feel good about yourself, while not putting pressure on yourself to do more.

CHAPTER ELEVEN

WHY SELF-IDENTITY MATTERS

Who do you want to be?

If you see yourself as someone who exercises, as a runner, a swimmer, a fit and strong person, you will naturally live up to these expectations of yourself. Conversely, if you see yourself as a lazy person, a bit of a loser perhaps, you will act exactly like a bit of a loser. Your identity is a self-fulfilling prophecy. So, what is your identity? How do you see yourself? Do you see yourself as strong or weak?

People who see themselves as 'a runner' or 'a triathlete' or 'a mountaineer' will seek out activities and a lifestyle that supports this version of themselves. They will go running or swimming or whatever, because that is who they are and what they do. They may not feel like it all the time, and they may have periods where they don't exercise, but they will return to it when the time is right. It's because that's who they are and that's how they see themselves.

Take a minute to think about how you see yourself. Do you have an image of yourself as a particular sort of person, or maybe as a bundle of different identities, depending on where you are and who you are with? Maybe you strongly identify with your job, or your role within a family. When you think about that person or collection of traits, is this who you want to be?

Do you see yourself as someone who is fit and active? It might not be part of your identity at the moment, but over time, it can be. You can become the person you want to be, you just have to want it. It's just a case of telling yourself that's who you are. Fake it until you make it.

Let's say you've decided you want to add in "I am fit and active" to how you see yourself. You want it to become part of you. The way to do this is just to behave like an active person would. What would a fit person do? Don't go emulating a top athlete who trains for four hours a day, instead all you need to do is to emulate the fitter version of yourself. So, if you were fitter, what would you do? What would that version of you be like? If I were fitter, I would make the time for a walk every day, I would do some stretches before bed, and I would choose the healthier option with food. Fit and healthy me would drink more water and go to bed at a more sensible time. I can't wave a magic wand and become someone else, but I can look at myself and think, what would a more motivated person do in my circumstances? Someone who sees themselves as an active person might choose to go for a bike ride at the weekend, rather than spending that time online shopping or baking a cake. Tiny changes will add up to a big change overall. Those little tweaks can become new habits, which will be much more effective than coming down the stairs one morning and declaring that you are going to overhaul your entire life. You don't have to change everything all at once. Try making one or two new habits that don't take long or aren't much effort. The fit and healthy me definitely does her stretches every night before bed. Those stretches might only take two minutes. But it all works towards being that person I want to be.

There are always trade-offs.

Sometimes we can be concerned about changing our identity because we worry about who we might become, and what might happen in our lives if we change what we do. This is completely normal and understandable. Even if we have habits we know are bad for us, we can be loath to lose those habits because of who we have become and what those habits give us. For example, some smokers can find it hard to give up smoking, not because they are addicted to the nicotine or the act of smoking itself, but because going out for a cigarette allows them a break from work, or any other situation they want to escape from. The highlight of their day is standing outside having a chat and a smoke with friends. By giving up smoking, they will no longer have that in their lives. Sometimes you have to look at what benefits you are getting from a negative situation. Perhaps you are actually gaining something from this lifestyle you say you want to change. Maybe you get more help from others because you put yourself in the role of a victim. Maybe people ask little of you because you are always telling them how bad things are. If you are thinking like this, it's useful to question whether you are unwittingly making sure nothing changes.

You may also have a bunch of people around you who you suspect might not be that supportive of you if you become healthier or more active. Again, this is really common. It's not just that they love you the way you are, it's that they don't want you holding up a mirror to their own behaviour and choices. If you get healthier and they don't, they may see it as a judgment on themselves—that you see yourself as somehow better than them, or that you have got a level of determination they lack. Maybe they make frequent disparaging comments, or little digs at people and you are worried that they might turn on you if you choose to mope less on the sofa moaning with them and go out for a walk instead. Even changing your moaning location from the sofa to the floor to create more movement could feel like inciting negative judgement: "Why are you sitting on the floor? What's wrong with you?" Sometimes it's simply that they are fearful of change, for you as well as for themselves. Maybe your family has always done things in a certain way and it's a bit of a stretch for some family members to cope with anything differing from the status quo.

This is a hard one. But it's about your identity. Who are you? Who do you want to be? Your friends and family will have to get over the fact that you have made some different life choices to them. In an ideal world, they will be supportive of you wanting to feel better and happier and taking some steps to achieve this. In reality, it might take them some time.

Change is scary, we tend to be risk averse, and it seems more comfortable to keep everything the same even when you're not happy with how things are. This is why it often takes a major life event for people truly to change their behaviour. A major health scare or losing something or someone important to you can be what it takes for you to realise that the worst has already happened, so there's nothing to lose from doing things differently.

Perhaps, when looking at your self-identity, you have noticed that you are constantly berating yourself for not being good enough. If only there were a switch where you could turn off that negative voice. You can work on silencing it by trying affirmations. These usually take the form of an "I am..." sentence that you repeat to yourself. It can be effective to say it as if it were already true, such as "I wake up motivated," or "I do not care what other people think". If you don't feel comfortable using the present tense, try saying "I will..." instead. When you have come up with a sentence that is personal to you, repeat it out loud or write it down. Acknowledge when you have achieved something that demonstrates the truth of your affirmation. For example, if you are using "I wake up motivated" or "I will wake up motivated" and today you did some stretches before breakfast, this shows that you *do* wake up motivated. Over time, repeating positive affirmations can help to overcome negative self-talk. It's all part of moving from a negative mindset into a more positive one. Here are a couple of common affirmations:

> *"Every day in every way, I am getting better and better."* Émile Coué

> *"I am strong, I am beautiful, I am enough."*

My personal favourite:

> *"I see pride! I see power! I see a bad-ass mother who don't take no crap off of nobody!"* Cool Runnings movie, 1993

It is not necessary to reinvent your entire life and personality. What I'm talking about is adding in a new, positive component to your identity, where you see yourself as somebody fit and strong, and as someone who enjoys moving their body. Little tweaks. Just imagine what that strong and active version of you would choose to do and what they would say to themselves.

CHAPTER TWELVE

CONFiDENCE AND COMFORT ZONES

Confidence and Fear of Failure

A lack of confidence and a fear of failure are annoyingly familiar and frustrating. Walking into a new environment like a gym or a club is daunting, especially if you don't look or feel the part. You might not have admitted to anyone that you are fearful of trying something new, but you certainly aren't alone.

That's why I propose starting really small with things you are comfortable with. You don't have to step right out of your comfort zone all at once. This is supposed to be a good thing, not a horrible scary thing. You can absolutely get fitter and move more without having to step foot in a gym, wear any Lycra, or even tell anyone else what you're doing.

It's worth examining what it is you are afraid of. If you can understand it, you can work around it. Most of us have a fear of being laughed at or talked about negatively. I'm an intensely private and shy person and will often avoid doing things I feel other people might notice. For example, I remember a recent absolutely stunningly beautiful clear winter's day. There was no wind and there was a tiny bit of warmth in the sun. I'd got it into my head that I really wanted to go in the sea—a bit of cold-water therapy is all the rage isn't it? So we went to the beach. I even had my swimsuit on under my clothes, but I chickened out of doing it. There were so many people walking on the beach and no one else was in the sea. The tide was right in so there wasn't much distance between the sea and the prom. I was nervous about how cold the sea would be anyway and couldn't bring myself to be seen in my swimsuit. I felt like everyone would point and laugh.

The fact is, I don't know what any of the other people on the beach would really have been thinking. They might have not even given me a second glance. I certainly wouldn't have taken up more than a few seconds of their thoughts. It's a terrible habit to ascribe negative thoughts to others, especially when I wouldn't think those thoughts myself. I know for a fact that if I'd seen someone else having a dip in the sea, I'd have thought, "Good for them! I wish I could do that." Maybe I'd have thought they were crazy, but it would be in an admiring rather than disparaging way. So why assume that everyone else around me is a horrible meanie?

Very few of us don't care what other people think of us and no one wants to feel like a fool. Shame is a powerful human emotion, and we try to avoid it.

But that's one of the brilliant things about being an absolute beginner in something. No one has any expectations of beginners. You're supposed to do it wrong. If you are looking to get back into fitness after a while off, consider trying something completely new. You'll have no preconceived ideas of your own ability based on what you used to do, and starting something new is fun. Also, if you've already committed to move more in your daily life, you will get fitter and more mobile quickly, so you should make fast progress in your new activity.

And yes, you might be nervous about trying something new, but this is a good thing and something to embrace.

A bit of stress on our system is actually good for us, as long as we relax again afterwards. Short-lived, rather than chronic stress, pushes your brain to be at its most alert and perform at its best. I'm talking about stress that pushes you gently and safely out of your comfort zone, like taking a test, making a speech, or getting to the top of a climbing frame (and back down again). It is a great way to build resilience and self-confidence. I'm sure you have done scary things in the past: you are a lot more resilient than you think you are.

Exercise puts your body under healthy stress when your muscles have to work. This is part of what gives us the benefits of exercise, as it's a short-term stressor which pushes our bodies to function well. Just like how your muscles grow back stronger after the stress of exercise, your mental resilience improves in the same way.

In doing something new that you are worried about, think of all the times in the past you've had to do this. Everything you do now had a first time. We all had first days at school, first days in a new job, first dates. They might not have all turned out to be wonderful, but where would you be now if you had never had a go? Acknowledge how brave you can be. If there's something you would really like to have a go at but haven't quite got the guts, how much better could your life be, how much more fun could you have, if you just tried it? If it doesn't work out, who cares? You can chalk it up to building resilience and proving to yourself that you are the sort of person who isn't afraid to try new things.

I really regret not getting into the sea the other day. You can tell, as I'm still banging on about it. Don't you find you kick yourself for the things you didn't do?

In Appendix 2, I have made a list of all the activities and sports I can think of that might give you a few ideas. I'm not suggesting that you have to do any of these as a regular thing. You might look at that list and think the whole thing is a big fat 'nope'. That's cool. But if you commit to moving more and getting the physical and mental benefits of exercise, you've got to do something, so what are you going to do?

I used to be intimidated by the idea of rock climbing. You go so horribly high up, and then what? You come back down again? Sounds pretty pointless. My husband Ross has been climbing since he was a teenager. I went with him once, had a massive freakout high on the wall and never went back. Then a new bouldering centre opened in our town. We live in a part of the country with no actual rocks at all, so this was a big deal to my climbing-obsessed husband. Bouldering, in case you don't know, is done without ropes, but on much shorter walls. It's still scary at the top, but it's not 'certain death if I fall' scary. More 'maybe broken ankle if I fall' - great! I gave it a go and soon got hooked. The atmosphere was so much friendlier and more inclusive than I'd found at other climbing places and our friend Guy came too, so I had a fellow newbie to hang out with.

Climbing is fun. I get to spend time with Ross and my friends. The people there are nice and it's a form of exercise I *actually want to do*. Ten years ago, I never would have seen myself getting into climbing. Never, ever.

Have an open mind about what you might like to do and grab opportunities to try new things.

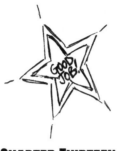

CHAPTER THIRTEEN

MOTIVATE YOURSELF

Should I reward myself for exercising?

So how are you going to get yourself to do more movement and exercise? Well, what about rewarding yourself? This is something that comes up fairly frequently, where the advice is usually along the lines of promise yourself a treat for doing the healthy thing. Does this work? Do rewards ever work as a motivator? The answer is sometimes, but probably not long term.

Let's say you promise yourself a takeaway if you go to the gym for an hour. The first, obvious, problem with this is that the reward isn't particularly healthy. Any food or drink-based reward will not be very good for you. Let's face it, if I promised myself an apple as a treat for going to the gym for an hour, it's not motivating in the slightest. Food-based rewards are problematic anyway. If I see unhealthy food as a reward, it's a slippery slope into 'treating' myself with food whenever something good or bad happens in my life. Good and bad things happen a lot, especially if you are looking for an excuse to treat yourself. While I don't count calories, I know that working out for an hour in the gym burns off way fewer calories than there are in a takeaway, and so if I'm looking to at least maintain my current weight, then I'm going to find that rewarding exercise with loads of calories will lead to negative consequences.

Another problem with using rewards for exercise is that I'm a grownup with my own money. I'm not a dog begging for a treat. There is no one else holding me accountable and telling me no, I can't have the new pair of shoes because I haven't been to the gym. I can afford the shoes and I want the shoes, so I'll just end up getting them anyway, whether I've been to the gym for an hour or not. If I had the willpower to say, "OK, I haven't been to the gym so I'm not getting the new shoes," I wouldn't be in this position in the first place. If I had the iron will to deny myself nice things or to do things I don't really want to do, then I'd be doing all the healthy stuff already.

Rewards work really well for training animals, but they don't work so well for humans. If the reward is big enough it could work. For example, if I said I will give you a million pounds if you exercise for an hour a day every day for a month, you'd magically find the time.

But if I said I'd give you a million pounds if you exercise for an hour every day for the next 30 years, would you still be able to do it? The reward is so far off it loses its attraction. But if I split those one million pounds over the 30 years (roughly) and said I'll give you £100 every day you exercise for an hour, maybe you would stick at it for quite a while? I think I would for £100 a day.

So, the reward has to be big enough and immediate enough to make it worth your while. Have you got anything you can reward yourself with that is really that motivating, that you wouldn't give yourself anyway and that you can realistically afford?

The trouble is, if someone offers you something as a reward, when the going gets tough you weigh up how much you actually want it. If it will not change your life and you can easily live without it, then it makes sense to abandon a task that is hard.

Once I've done a few months of exercising for an hour a day, if I'm only doing it for the money, I'd soon be well off from my £100 a day and the reward would lose its power. I would question whether I really needed the money. It would be the money rather than the exercise itself which would be the deciding factor.

However, maybe the reward could be a short-term thing that would be enough to keep you going for long enough to help the exercise become a habit. It could be an upcoming holiday or other event you want to be fit for. But there has to come a point where the desire to do the thing, in this case exercise, switches from being motivated by external factors to something internal. If the exercise is something you just want to do, you don't have to decide if the reward is worth the effort.

Praise is reward too, so if you're going to run a marathon simply to get a load of likes from your social media followers, you are being motivated by the praise, not because you actually want to put yourself through all that running. There will come a point when you weigh up whether those likes are worth it.

On the other hand, you probably know people who have achieved extraordinary things, and you have no idea why they persevered with it. It's because their intrinsic motivation was strong. There was something inside driving them, even if people around them were telling them to stop, or if their circumstances seemed really difficult. You have got to find the thing inside that is going to motivate you, no matter what.

What drives you?

No one ever regretted getting strong. There really is nothing like it. How do you want to feel? Strong and capable, or weak and flabby? Whatever your age, gender, shape or size, you can feel strong.

My version of strong is different from yours, but I'm guessing we both want to feel stronger than we do now. As a 40-year-old woman, I see perimenopause on the horizon and I know how important it is for women to maintain their strength as they age. Improving your strength is good for your bone density, protecting it against osteoporosis. Muscle strength will also help compensate for any weaknesses in joints as you get older, keeping you mobile. A big motivator for me, now, is to get into good habits that I hope will last me into old age and keep me active and healthy as long as possible. I want to stay free from bad backs, knees, etc now, so that those niggles don't turn into chronic pain when I'm older. That's my long-term motivation.

In the medium term, I want to be fit to be prepared. I want to be physically ready for whatever life throws at me. I don't know what's going to happen. The world is a strange and unpredictable place, so I want to be fit enough to cope with it. For me, that involves a mix of strength and endurance activities. I want to be strong enough to climb over a fence or carry my child somewhere. If there's no fuel, which doesn't seem that outlandish these days, I want to be physically able to walk or cycle wherever I might need to go. I also want to be capable enough perhaps to chop down a (small) tree and collect the wood for a fire. These are things that our ancestors wouldn't have baulked at, as it would have been their daily life. I might never *need* to use my body in such a way, but there are plenty of non-emergency situations when a bit of fitness comes in useful. For example, that country walk where you somehow get completely lost and end up miles from where you should be. You need the reserves to keep going until you can find a road. Or the shopping trip where you walk into town and end up unexpectedly buying several large items that you then have to carry home.

For me, fitness is all about being prepared. Can I run? Can I walk a long way? Can I carry heavy stuff? Can I climb my way out of somewhere?

You might want to include "can I fight?" as a question to add to the above list. Humans are a very violent species, after all. My preference is to be fit enough to run away, but you might consider being able to fight as a life skill. I'm not going to go into depth on this, as it's not for everyone and my focus is about stuff you can do at home or with minimal outside training. However, if it appeals to you, there are many martial arts, from Eastern to Western, modern to historical, armed and unarmed, and they make a valuable addition to your mental and physical health. There are plenty of mental benefits to training in martial arts - it won't make you a more violent individual, quite the opposite, in fact.

What do you want to be fit for? This is completely personal to you. It motivates me to want to be strong and have energy. For me, the desire to be physically strong and fit in the medium and long term provides my intrinsic motivation. It has nothing to do with any reward or anything anybody else might say to me or encourage me to do.

Last summer, my husband and I had a rare afternoon and evening off without the kids. It was a beautiful day and we had booked a table at a lovely country pub. We decided to go for a walk beforehand. About 4 miles in, I looked at the route and how much time we had until our table reservation and realised that we would not make it to the pub on time at our current pace. Keen not to miss out on food, I thought I could see a different path on the map that looked shorter, so we took that. After another mile, I looked at our location and realised that we were actually still on the original route and as we were almost halfway, we might as well carry on. So, we ran. We covered the next 6 miles at a swift pace, with a mix of jogging and brisk walking. It was actually quite fun, and fortunately we had a laugh rather than a massive argument. In the end, we made it to the pub with enough time to change our sweaty clothes. The burger and pint in the riverside pub garden tasted even more amazing, knowing that I'd just walked and jogged 11 miles to get it. Having a base level of fitness meant that I could go beyond my normal limits without too much discomfort and even enjoy it. I was tired for a day or two afterwards, but it is one of my best memories of that summer.

Motivation for the here and now: four ways that work

By now, you might be starting to feel like you want to move more. Perhaps you are motivated to make exercise part of your life. However, just thinking about it will not get you anywhere. I believe that to stop procrastinating you need to pinpoint your motivation and focus on how doing this cycle/swim/walk will make you *feel*. Focusing on feelings is helpful for stopping overthinking and talking yourself out of it.

Your brain hasn't been helping you until now, so let's try to get the thinking part out of the equation. Instead, can you imagine any good feelings that you will get from exercising? With a little imagination you can really boost your motivation through these four areas:

1. Knowing how it'll make you feel

2. Discipline and habit

3. Visualising your end goal

4. Other people

1. Let's start with knowing how it'll make you feel:

There are many ways of being motivated to do something. You could be motivated to do something because the act itself is pleasurable, like a walk in the countryside on a sunny day. You enjoy the walk while you're doing it and you feel you could just keep walking all day.

You could be motivated by the satisfaction you know you will get afterwards, for example, pushing yourself to run further than you ever have before. You know that if you push yourself, you will achieve something great, and the self-satisfaction afterwards is well worth the discomfort.

You can also be motivated by knowing how you will feel physically afterwards, like the mysterious 'runner's high', or having pleasantly tired muscles you know are getting stronger. Flexing your arm and feeling your 'guns', or moving your foot up and down and seeing your calf muscle expand and contract is great. As I've already said, there's no better feeling than feeling strong and physically powerful.

It can be very tempting for an over-thinker like me to decide I'm going to start a new exercise regime and then spend an inordinate amount of time researching what I'm going to do and making a plan—preferably a spreadsheet, and preferably using different colours for different categories. That genuinely makes me happy. But moving my body is not an academic exercise—if it were I'd be super fit! By making it all about thinking and analysing and coming up with plans, I'm doing the very opposite of what I need to be doing and setting myself up to fail. A pretty spreadsheet is not actually that motivating, as it was making the spreadsheet that was enjoyable, rather than the exercise itself.

It takes time to make a new habit, and with exercise, you need to commit to something for at least six weeks for the habit to stick. Six weeks is a long time if you're not enjoying it, so you need to find whatever aspect of the activity that motivates you. Do you enjoy the activity itself? Does it feel fun at the time? Do you enjoy the feeling of satisfaction from having achieved something difficult? Or do you enjoy how your body feels afterwards? If you can find something that gives you all three, then you're on to a winner.

The thing you enjoy may not be something you can do every day. If skiing turns out to be the thing that you absolutely love and crave, but you live in Norfolk, you can still use skiing as the hook. Everything you do, every move you make, is training. You are training to be a better skier even in one of the flattest parts of the country. Skiers need strong legs, and good balance. Those are things you can work on wherever you are, even with no equipment at all. By keeping in mind how utterly wonderful it feels to go skiing, the freedom of the slopes, the sun on your face, the powdery snow, the magnificent views, you will find yourself much more willing and able to keep yourself moving the rest of the year so that when you hit the slopes, it'll be a breeze. And no spreadsheet is necessary.

2. Forming habits

Habits are things we do without having to plan or make a special effort to do. They just happen. When we think about forming new habits, we tend to assume that the new habit has got to be something big and noticeable, like saying you're going to go to the gym three days a week. But when you think about the habits you have already, even the bad habits, like biting your nails or staying up too late, they are actually pretty small things. Biting my nails takes me seconds at a time - I don't sit down to spend an hour a day biting my nails, or schedule in special 'biting time' three days a week. Gross. But the small nibbles here and there add up to pretty awful looking nails, without me even realising that I've done it.

Similarly, I clean my teeth twice a day because it's a habit. I clean my teeth whether or not I'm actively feeling motivated, it's just what I do. More conscious effort goes into the teeth cleaning than the nail biting, but it is something I cannot imagine going through the day without doing.

We can take this approach to adding more movement into our lives. Instead of grand gestures, we should think instead about those few minutes here and there. If a few seconds of biting my nails can have a significant effect, so can moving more throughout the day. If movement is a part of my day in the same way as cleaning my teeth, it'll become something I don't even have to be motivated to do.

I've fallen into the trap of deciding I'm going to start a new fitness regime by going to the gym for an hour three days a week, failing to consider that life is made up of tiny habits and routines. Something that takes maybe an hour at a time is more than just a single habit - there are all the other routines that you have got to alter to fit in that hour of exercise. Few of us have a free hour in the day just sitting there waiting to be filled. Even if it's TV watching time that you feel you can re-use as gym time, that TV time is probably a habit and part of your daily schedule. By going to the gym instead, you are not just gaining gym time; you are also losing TV time, which you'll either want to make up elsewhere by staying up later, or you'll just have to accept that you will not get to watch TV. In effect, by making a new habit, you must break old ones at the same time. Which, unless the new habit is more enjoyable than the old one, is hard.

From what scientists are telling us about movement and exercise, an important factor seems to be frequency. Little and often is ideal. I suggest that if we want to be more active, which involves making new habits, we should do this by incorporating it into existing habits and routines as much as possible. This means we are only adding in, rather than having to take away as well. So, add some movement into your TV time by sitting on the floor, doing some stretches, making sure you get up during ad breaks or between episodes. If you added tiny bits of movement into your normal daily activities, how much additional movement could you get into your day? Those minutes spent brushing teeth could also be spent standing on one leg or doing slow squats.

It still takes awareness and discipline to create new habits, but by "stacking your life" as Katy Bowman puts it - adding movement into your normal activities - it is much more achievable than having to break existing habits at the same time.

To stop myself biting my nails, I paint them. I don't want to eat nail varnish, and I don't want the varnish to look all chipped either. Telling myself not to bite my nails doesn't work. I need to stop myself in a way that doesn't require will power. Having to use will power is where we've been going wrong with trying and failing to get more exercise. What works much better is putting the factors in place that will make it harder to do the things we don't want to do, and easier to do the things we know we ought to do . Probably one of the best examples of this would be to get a dog, especially one that will look at you pleadingly with the lead in its mouth. I don't have a dog, but I do have kids. The kids don't want to exercise, but seeing them sitting all day in front of screens irritates me enough that I will force them out for some form of exercise and I go too.

When you are sitting at your desk, make sure you have a large glass of water (or a big mug of tea or whatever you like to drink) in front of you. If it's there, you're likely to drink it. And if you drink it, eventually you're going to have to get up because you'll need the toilet. In this situation, all you have had to remember to do is take a big drink to your desk. You haven't had to tell yourself to get up and move - something you don't want to do because you are absorbed in your work. Instead, your bladder has done the motivating work for you.

I've already talked about not getting changed to do exercise. The less we think of it as a special, 'other' activity, the better. It is so much easier to do a few squats when waiting for a pan of water to boil, than it is to have to get changed, get in the car and go to a gym to do those same squats as part of a gym session. You could do all the same exercises over the course of a day that you could do in half an hour at the gym. There's no law that says that strength training has to be done all at once. Your muscles don't know the difference anyway.

Remove the barriers that are making movement harder to do, such as having to travel, having to get changed, having to fit to someone else's timetable, and you've made the good habit much more achievable than it was before.

3. Visualisation: The power of imagination

We humans have incredible imaginations. We can imagine ourselves into all sorts of stressful situations that haven't happened and probably won't. I've had many a difficult conversation *in my head* with a friend I've fallen out with, or a boss who won't listen to me. The reality of the situation is never as dramatic or interesting as the one I've played out beforehand, or the one I have in my head afterwards, when I think of all the devastatingly witty and cutting things I should have said.

In a new relationship I'm sure that you gave the person you barely knew all sorts of characteristics that later turned out not to belong to them at all. Maybe they weren't as funny or clever or trustworthy as you imagined them to be. Even if you don't feel you are that creative in your thinking, I'm sure you can think of somewhere you would rather be, or where you would like to go on your dream holiday. We can use our imaginations as a tool. In fact, it has been studied in some depth that if you can really imagine yourself doing exercise and training your muscles, or learning to play a piece on the piano, for example, the same areas of your brain fire up as if they were actually doing the exercise or playing the piano. You can train your brain to learn a new skill, without even moving, as long as you imagine it really hard.

Great, you think. I can sit in my armchair and imagine I'm running a mile and that will count. Well, no, it won't, I'm afraid. To get the benefits of exercise, you have to exercise. However, we can use our imagination to help.

If I'm working on a difficult route at the climbing gym, one that has a scary move that I can't quite get my body to agree to do, I will visualise myself doing it for days afterwards. I will teach myself how it is supposed to feel and I will do that move over and over again in my head. When I get back in the climbing centre, it may not feel in reality much like I imagined it, but I am fired up to get on that wall and have a go. If you can visualise doing the activity you want to do, whether it's a single climbing move, the route you're going to cycle, or lifting a heavy weight, you will find that the more you visualise it and the more detail you can imagine, the more you will want to do it for real. Imagine not just what it's going to look like, but the sounds, the smells, and the physical sensations you will experience.

Another way I use my imagination to help my motivation to exercise is something I've done ever since I was a child. As a child, I read a lot of fantasy books, with plenty of adventure and danger and swashbuckling. When I was out and about, in my head I was on a quest. To the untrained eye, you may have seen an unremarkable-looking girl riding a bicycle down a track, but actually you were witnessing Aragorn, or Robin Hood, off on a mission and trying to escape their enemies. These days, I rarely pretend to be Robin Hood, though it would make woodland walks a lot more fun if I did. I'm more likely to pretend I'm on a challenge of some sort, perhaps a TV programme where I have to beat the other contestants to the goal. You might think I've lost the plot, but it's in the confines of my head—or it was—and can make a rather mundane walk a bit more exciting.

If you are trying to find the motivation to exercise, focusing on how it makes you feel, and using your imagination are really helpful tools that will boost that intrinsic drive, or desire, to get moving. However, by far the best way I've found to make exercise a part of your life is to do it with others.

4. Get social

As I already mentioned in the earlier section on how we evolved, we are social creatures and need to cooperate with others for our society to work. Nearly all the best things in our lives happen with others. Even the most introverted of us need some social connection. Yes, there are some genuine hermits and some people who would really rather be left completely alone, but they are the exception rather than the rule. Most of us like to spend time around others, even if we then retreat to our caves for a bit of alone time.

Have you ever been to a concert or a sports match, where the crowd is singing and dancing as one? It's the most incredibly joyous feeling to be part of something like that. Activities such as Parkrun, Christmas Day swims, cycling groups, etc, all exist because it's much more fun to splash about in the North Sea in December with others as mad as you, than it is to go down to chilly, grey Felixstowe on your own and have a dip. We feel safer in a group with others looking out for us, and the camaraderie and competitiveness will ensure you push yourself more than if you were on your own.

Have you got any friends or family members who also want to get fitter? If you can exercise together, that's brilliant. If they live too far away, you can still create a virtual group. I am part of a WhatsApp group of four who all do yoga. We message each other when we've done a good session or need a bit of motivation from the group. It's a friendly reminder when a message pops up from someone that I should do some yoga today.

Taking part in organised group activities can give you much more of a buzz than simply doing it on your own. For example, Parkrun is well established as being good for people's mental health. Yes, you could do a 5km run or walk on your own on a Saturday morning, but going and doing that 5km as part of a big, encouraging, enthusiastic group will leave you feeling happier for other reasons as well just the workout. And you will get to see other people who are at the same level as you. Even if you are walking at the back, there will be someone else right there with you. You won't be the only one. And if you have the smallest competitive bone in your body, you'll be motivated to practice during the week so that you're a bit faster by the time the next social walk/run/swim/cycle comes around.

Goals and Challenges

Goals can be uninspiring if they are not really your goals and you are just setting them because you think you ought to. If you've come across goal setting over the years at school or work, you know that they aren't often that motivating if you're told to make them when you don't really want to.

The question is, how willing are you to do things differently? How willing are you, really, to change up your usual routine? That is ultimately going to be the deciding factor in whether you succeed. You won't change anything if you keep doing what you have always done. If you're setting yourself a goal because you feel you ought to, but it's something you don't really want to do, or you're never going to have the time, don't bother. Save yourself the inevitable feelings of failure and disappointment and be realistic right from the start. Instead, what could be some small wins for you? It could be something as small as every week trying a new vegetable you never normally cook with, or going for a quick walk around the block every evening after dinner.

Where I think goals or challenges have a place is when they are ones that life naturally throws at you, which you can take advantage of, such as an upcoming major birthday or a holiday. If it's something that's going to happen, you can use this to your advantage to give you motivation to get started. Imagine how good you'll feel on holiday being able to walk up and down the steep steps to the beach without having to stop and pant halfway up. This is not some arbitrary goal you've set yourself that makes no difference to your life whether or not you achieve it. It is something that will make a tangible improvement to your enjoyment of your trip to the beach.

There are also very motivating challenges you can do as part of a team. In December, some friends and I take part in a challenge called *Run Up To Christmas*, which is a charity event where you set yourself a goal distance and then, individually or as a team, you have from 1st–25th December to hit the distance by running or walking. My husband and I do the challenge with friends who live in France, so we can't do any of it together, but we track what we do on the website, and we chat about it in a messenger group. It's highly motivating for several reasons:

1. There's the target we want to hit.

2. There's the camaraderie of being in a group,

so you've got others to spur you on when you aren't in the mood.

3. There's the competition element. Two of us have a bit of an unspoken competition about who's going to 'win', i.e., get the most miles. We're far too nice to be open about it, but we both know it's competitive. This year we were pretty much neck and neck until I lost a couple of days because of illness and she got an unassailable lead. Next year though...

4. Being part of a wider group challenge that is organised by someone else means you pay an entry fee, so you have made a commitment from the start, and they use emails and social media to help jolly you along.

It is important to incorporate more movement into your daily routine in an enjoyable way that improves your life, rather than adding on an extra layer of pressure. Challenges and goals are like the icing on the cake if you feel you want to do a little more or add a bit of extra motivation, but they are not essential.

You won't be motivated all the time

Motivation is a feeling like all others. There are going to be days, weeks, months even, where you lack motivation. Just like you wouldn't expect to feel any other emotion consistently throughout your life, the same applies to motivation. It's OK to take time out. Shit happens. This is also where those little movement habits you have made will come into their own.

The problem is that the less you move, the less you feel like moving. So, if you don't feel like exercising but you know you need to, sometimes you just have to get up and do something. Change your mental state by changing your physical state. It really works. Take yourself out of your head and into your body. Tell yourself you're just going to go for a ten-minute walk and get out the door. If, after three minutes, you really want to turn round and go home, then you've still done six minutes. You might find that once you're out, you want to keep going a little longer. Or set a timer and tell yourself you're going to spend five minutes dancing, or doing exercises, or walking up and down the stairs. It could be something really random that entertains you: why not spend five minutes rolling around on the floor or swinging your arms about? There's no right or wrong. Don't get changed, don't waste any time on preparation or you won't get started at all. It doesn't really matter what you do. If you do something so silly you make yourself laugh, all the better. Don't take yourself too seriously. Just spend five minutes moving your body around. Notice whether your mental state has changed afterwards. Do you still feel so feeble?

If five minutes isn't possible for you, put the kettle on or do a small task. While you're waiting for the kettle to boil, or when you've done your task, start swinging your arms, circle them around, bend forward, do a star jump, any sort of movement that feels good to you. See how it feels to do something, anything.

If you're not up to doing anything self-directed, find yourself a ten-minute workout or yoga session on YouTube. Get someone else to tell you what to do and just follow along. Depending on your personality, you might find it easier to be given instructions, or you might want to just do your own thing. Start with the action and the motivation will follow.

CHAPTER FOURTEEN

STARTING BEFORE YOU ARE READY

Have you ever told yourself you'll start something on a certain date? That you can't start a new fitness regime until the New Year, or until after the summer holidays? It's better just to start now, whenever now is.

On the 23rd December 2021, I was feeling really low. The autumn had been a series of Covid-related inconveniences. Nothing major, but nearly two years of pandemic worry had ground me down. I had also had a pretty strong reaction to the booster vaccine, and I had felt rough for a week. Christmas was nearly here, and I wasn't feeling festive—we were isolating at home and dreading taking the final lateral flow that would tell us whether we could spend Christmas Day with our family, or whether that was going to be yet another nice thing cancelled. I had no energy at all. I tried doing a few stretches and ended up lying on my back next to the Christmas tree, having a bit of a cry. I just felt so down. I wanted to move, I knew I ought to, but I couldn't bring myself to.

My husband came in and was obviously pretty concerned about the state I was in. I explained how pathetic and flabby I was feeling and how I hated feeling like this.

"Right, we're going to do a workout now," he said. I reluctantly agreed, even though I didn't think I'd do much. We put on some music, he went and got his dumbbells and my kettlebell, and we set a timer for 20 minutes. I figured I'd do four different exercises, repeated over the 20 minutes and I'd rest when I wanted to. It turned out to be a surprisingly good workout, especially since I had done nothing like it for as long as I could remember, doing push-ups and squats and planks and lifting the kettlebell up with one arm. I had gone from lying on the floor in a heap to doing proper exercise without even thinking about it. All we did was set the timer, put on the music, and get on with it.

We carried on doing the 20-minute workouts most days over the Christmas period. It took a bit of trial and error with the exercises, but I usually chose four different ones that used different muscles. I did 12 reps of each exercise but rested when I wanted for as long as I wanted. Some exercises required a kettlebell or dumbbells, and some just used my bodyweight.

The most amazing thing about that first workout on 23rd December was how much better I felt afterwards. I can't overstate it. My entire outlook on life changed. I didn't feel like crying any more and I didn't feel weak any more. I felt fresher and happier and energised. It's such a cliché and something I'd heard fitness freaks go on about in the past, but I'd never had a noticeable effect from exercise before. I guess it's a bit like people who witness a miracle and become religious converts. You can't believe it until you've experienced it for yourself.

I have to say, though, that I never would have done that workout unless my husband had done it with me. Left to my own devices, I probably would have stayed on the floor until I got too cold. Since then, when I said I wasn't in the mood to do the workout, he didn't push me and he often used it as an excuse not to do it either, so it doesn't always work. But we got started. We didn't wait until the New Year, and so we got a week's worth of exercising done that wouldn't have happened otherwise. And I got a week of feeling better, which is the most important thing of all.

Don't wait for the time to be right, for the conditions to be perfect, or for your motivation to peak. Just get on and do something. Take yourself by surprise and see what you can do.

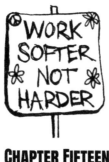

CHAPTER FIFTEEN

WORK SOFTER NOT HARDER

'Just work harder' is a mantra for so many and our prevailing Western protestant work ethic means many of us feel we ought to do something useful at all times. Feel you're failing at life? It's because you're just not working hard enough. The people we hold up as inspirational examples are those that have picked themselves up by their bootstraps, overcome massive adversity, and made it despite the odds. They didn't sit around eating biscuits and relaxing, they got out there and did it, whatever 'it' is.

But the flip-side of this is that we are taught to ignore the cues our bodies are giving us, not to listen when we're tired or have had enough, and to just keep pushing, pushing, pushing. We're all about carrying on and not giving up. Work culture encourages us to work beyond our contracted hours and to always be available. The person who walks in the door at 9am sharp and walks out at bang on 5pm is not considered a team player and is probably not promotion material.

There's no point at which work is finished, because you can always work harder. There's always more you can do.

Do you feel it's your duty, or an expectation you place on yourself, to do as much as you can, whether that's making money, helping others, or living a fulfilling life? How many of us can maintain that sort of pace indefinitely? We need to listen to what our bodies are telling us. If you are living at full steam ahead and at your limit, it's no wonder you don't have any energy or space in your life for movement and physical activity.

If we can let go of the expectations we place on ourselves so that we no longer feel that we have to be productively maximising every second of available time, this can lead us to be at peace with the idea of not getting everything done. Or not appearing to get everything done. A gentle amble round the block may seem on the surface not to be very productive - that's time you could spend working or doing something 'useful' - but in fact it is important time. If you need to label this wandering around time as something, label it as 'self-care' or good for your physical and mental health. But in fact, the most radical thing you could do would be not to categorise it as anything at all.

Yes, life is short, and we should make the most of it. But also, the world is absolutely batshit crazy. If everyone just calmed down and took it easier, maybe the world would be a better place. Maybe if our leaders went for more strolls around their local area they would be more in touch with the world, with nature, and with their fellow humans.

With fitness, and our usual mindsets of work, work, work, it's easy to become demoralised when the results we want don't appear straight away. Whenever I take up running (again) after a break, I can get hugely frustrated that I'm back to square one, and it takes weeks of consistent effort to get to the point where I can jog for ten minutes without stopping. Running a whole 5K in one go takes me months of training.

This is the problem with being too goal-oriented with fitness. We become impatient to reach the goal and then demoralised when it seems so far away. When our mindset is one that is about working harder to achieve goals, and our self-esteem is based on achievement, the people who are most likely to succeed are the ones who are naturally good at fitness.

With exercising and movement, success doesn't have to mean pushing yourself to the point of exhaustion or punishing your body until it breaks. Instead, why not take a more intuitive approach? Choose how you are going to move depending on how you are feeling.

Feeling sad or low? Try dancing to some energising music or exercising with a friend. If no friend is available, how about going for a walk while phoning a friend or listening to a comedy podcast?

Feeling irritable, angry, or frustrated? Lift some heavy weights to some heavy music, punch a punchbag, run up a hill, or dive into a cool swimming pool.

Feeling tired? Just head out for a walk, with no expectation of how far you're going to go. See how you feel when you get out. Or try an online yoga workout that describes itself as relaxing or restorative. Or how about not doing anything at all, and just lie on the floor and do a bit of the breathing described in chapter nine. If, once you're down there, you feel like doing a bit of stretching, then have a go at that.

When I have tried to get back into exercise in the past, I've gone online and downloaded a plan, or devised my own, where I'm supposed to do certain workouts on certain days and rest on, say, Tuesdays and Sundays. The problem is that things come up; you have a dreadful night's sleep, or you miss a workout for some other reason, or two or three. Before you know it, you are well and truly off the wagon and watching it roll off into the sunset while you slump on the side of the road, feeling like you've failed. Nowadays, I prefer a more relaxed approach to when I'm going to exercise and what I'm going to do. It means I don't do as much as I could of certain things that I don't enjoy, and over the years I end up having phases of one thing then another, but at least I'm consistent in doing *something*. If I only feel like walking, I go for a walk, rather than thinking, well today's the day I should do a HIIT workout, but I really don't feel up to that today so I'm going to sit on the sofa eating crisps instead. By listening to my body, it means I am more in tune with it.

Happiness is found along the way

Another issue I have with the whole 'just work harder' philosophy is that it presumes that there is an end point you are going to reach. You work harder and harder until you achieve... something. You make a million-pound deal, you win the ultramarathon, you get promoted. But does the ultramarathon runner win their race and then retire? Of course not. They then set themselves an even more outrageous target, like running five ultramarathons in five days. And when they've achieved that they move onto something else. (I'm looking at you, Rich Roll. Check him out, it's an inspiring story, but he's definitely one of the 'work harder' brigade.) You don't see Richard Branson or Elon Musk retiring to a cottage in the country with a few chickens, do you? They can't stop, they are always onto the next project or challenge. With people like that, I believe it is the challenge that makes them happy. The challenge itself motivates them; they derive pleasure from working towards something. But if you are miserably working hard to reach a fitness goal with the belief that when you reach it you will be happy, please stop and think whether this is really the case. It's like when people work hard to earn enough money to buy their dream house, because everything will be better when they move to the country. When they finally get their dream house, yes, they feel amazing for a bit, but they soon fall back into feeling as dissatisfied as they were before. Just like lottery winners do. If you were unhappy before you got the thing you were working for, you are likely to be unhappy after you get it. You are still the same person, just with better stuff.

Who do you need the success for, anyway? Is it for yourself, or for other people's admiration, respect, or love? How strongly do you feel the need to post about your achievements on social media?

When you are getting into exercise, it's a fallacy to think that once you have run the London Marathon or climbed the mountain that you will have 'won' exercise. You can't get to a certain level of fitness and then stop. The gains you've made won't just stay there, it's not like reaching a certain level of XP in a video game. You don't get to be a Level 50 runner and stay Level 50 even if you stop running. You'll pretty soon be back at Level 3 or 4.

If exercise is purely a means to an end, it's going to make you miserable. It's going to be another thing to 'just work harder' at, to keep pushing yourself and overriding what your body wants to do, in service of some end goal that may never come. It's absolutely imperative that if you want to find joy in movement and exercise that you focus on the here and now, the 'journey', rather than the end goal.

For someone who isn't a natural athlete, and who will never win a medal in anything or appear to achieve anything that the outside world would consider worthy of celebration, we have to let go of the idea that fitness is about working harder and harder until we achieve something. We have to be patient and find enjoyment from the movement itself, rather than the kudos we might get from reaching a target.

The Hardest Part

What's the hardest part of exercising? Is it the first 100 metres of the run? The last mile?

The hardest part of exercise is getting up out of your chair and getting started. If you can do that, you're winning.

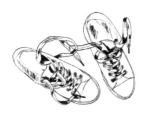

CHAPTER SIXTEEN

WHEN I'M NINETY-NINE

We need to move more. It's a fact. Being sedentary most of the time is simply not enough physical activity to give you the mental and physical benefits of exercise.

If the benefits of movement were put into a pill, we would all be taking it every day, as we would feel happier and more positive. Our immune systems would work better so we would get less sick, less often. Our bodies would work more effectively and efficiently—our digestion would work better, we would have a better sex life, we would sleep better and wake feeling more refreshed. Our weight would be more stable. When it's written on paper, it's an easy decision that we need to move more. There are no downsides, no negative side effects, and honestly, it can be enjoyable too.

Unfortunately, over the years, we have designed out the need to move as much as possible. We're not quite at the Wall-E stage yet, but if you have a desk-based job, you probably don't need to move your body much at all. We shuffle from one supportive chair to another throughout the day.

You'll know if you're not moving enough. If you get out of puff climbing the stairs or make that involuntary groan getting up out of a chair. If you feel so tired but can't switch off to go to sleep at night, or if you just feel low or down quite a lot, for no particular reason, then it's possible you need to get moving.

Human beings are capable of quite extraordinary physical feats. We are endurance masters, and yet the vast majority of us never test our limits and see what we could be physically capable of if we got to peak condition. That's something that other people do. But all of us possess the potential. The equipment is sitting there unused, and we're a bit miserable and a bit fat, and we know we're not making the best use of our lives. When you were a small child, I bet you loved to move. You probably couldn't sit still and were always running about, climbing trees, being a ninja or a horse or a fairy.

But you've grown up to hate exercise? That's ok, I did too. I cannot stand competitive sport. Exercise can be really boring, time-consuming, and expensive. And when we have competing priorities and things we would rather do, putting on some sportswear and voluntarily doing something uncomfortable falls way down the list.

However, fitness doesn't have to be about punishing yourself on a treadmill for hours at a time. The important thing is to move as much as possible throughout the day and get outside into some green space at least once a week, if not more. You don't have to exert yourself to exhaustion to get fitter. You can get the benefits by choosing to do gentle, everyday movements; by going for a brisk walk, and just from getting up from your chair. Build it into your day and be intentional about it. Notice the muscles you are using when doing different activities, be that pushing a trolley around the supermarket, carrying the shopping bags, scrubbing the kitchen worktop, running to catch the train or bus. It's all movement and it all counts.

There will be times when you move less. Life has a way of throwing these curveballs at us. The key is to accept that it happens, that nobody's perfect or perfectly motivated all the time, and allow it. Just get back to it when you can and do what is doable at the moment. Something will spark a glimmer of motivation, so seize it and take action.

Become a person who moves. Make being active part of your identity—it's who you are as a human, so own it. There are so many ways of moving that are enjoyable. Movement is like the food you eat; it is that essential to life. Exercise or training is like the treats: nice to have and make life more interesting, but not essential in large portions if you are getting a balanced movement diet. Keep yourself accountable by working towards a goal that you really want to achieve, join a group or create your own.

You will never be at the point where you are fully ready to start, so don't keep putting it off until you reach some mythical point in time where there is literally nothing else to do, the stars align and you get a magical burst of energy from on high. Start now. Actually now. Just get up and move your arms and legs around, put on some great music and just move. There are no rules. It doesn't matter what you do. If no one knows what you are doing, they can't tell you that you're doing it wrong. You don't have to join a club or do a specific form of exercise. It's your body. You know what feels good to you. We all have to start somewhere, so just start by focusing on what feels good. Don't get hung up on what you ought to do, what you ought to look like, or what someone your age/gender ought to be doing. This is all about you. It's your body, your mental and physical health, your life.

Imagine yourself at the age of 99 looking back on your life and the things you did with it. You can't live it for anyone else or through anyone else. You are the only one who knows what it feels like to be you. It is up to you to be good to your body, to look after it and nurture it so that you are as prepared as possible to cope with whatever life throws at you, and also have some fun along the way.

Appendix 1: Your Fitness Plan

In chapter fifteen I warned about the dangers of making and breaking plans, but if you find it helpful to get something on paper, this is the time and the place. You will see that the template I propose can be as vague as you like. The most important part is the 'Why' column, so you know exactly why you have written something on your plan and how it will benefit you.

Despite having produced an example plan, I am not trying to tell you what to do. If I did, you wouldn't stick to it because it wouldn't be meaningful to you. This is your chance to discover what is going to work in your life.

There are things to consider in writing your plan: what you feel you need to do to be fit enough; what you are actually motivated to build into your daily life; and what you have time for.

Let's look at time first. Go back to chapter three to look at the different ways of incorporating movement into your day that don't add much in the way of additional time. How can you tweak your current habits and activities to add movement? Can you schedule short movement breaks into your sedentary time?

In terms of the specific activities you need to do, head back to chapter one for details of what sort of exercise you need to be doing to be 'fit enough'. You can look to build up to around 150 minutes of activity each week with a mix of strength and endurance. There is an example of how you could break this down in the example below.

Finally, consider what you enjoy and what you are motivated to do. This is the most important factor in making your plan. If you like doing something, are motivated to do it and it gives you pleasure, then you will be able to find some time to do it. Chapter twelve on rewards and motivation might help you here.

An Example Plan

See below for a draft plan with some examples. The 'movement throughout the day' section should have the most entries. This is how you are going to make small, sustainable changes to get more movement into your life.

In this example plan, most of the movement comes from the everyday stuff – the squatting instead of bending down, the standing on one leg, etc. Then there are some small sessions of actual strength training to get a bit more moderate intensity into the week. For endurance, there's a Sunday morning swim and a country walk some time at the weekend. I've gone for the full 150 minutes here so you can see what it might look like, but this is not me saying that this is what you have to do. If you are starting from scratch, please don't feel you need to fill in 150 minutes' worth of activities from the get-go. Remember, anything you do that is more than what you are already doing is fantastic. You might start off with one two-minute strength workout and change absolutely nothing else.

There is an additional section at the end of the plan for 'How do I feel now?' This is to give you a snapshot of how you feel about your strength, energy level and motivation. How physically strong do you feel, how much energy have you got, and how motivated are you to move? Don't overthink it when scoring, it's just a quick overview which you can then use later on as a comparison.

There is a blank version of this plan and more examples of daily movement which you can download at www.easyfitnessforquitters.com.

Movement throughout the day

What	When	How	Why
Sit on the floor when watching TV	Every evening, for at least half an hour.	Put a cushion on the floor and sit on it or lie on it.	Have to use core muscles to support myself, more movement as it's less comfortable, use leg muscles to get up and down from the floor.
Stand on one leg when cleaning teeth	Twice a day	One minute standing on each leg while brushing	Works core muscles, improves strength and balance
Squat instead of bend to pick up items	Any time – many times per day		Builds strength in leg and bum muscles.
Daily walking	Every school day	Walking my daughter to school	Total 40 minutes of walking.

Specific strength-building

What	When	How	Why
Yoga	Twice a week – one morning and once at the weekend	Follow a 20 minute video on YouTube	Improve strength and flexibility
Ten minute strength routine	Monday and Friday lunchtime	Ten reps each of squats, lunges and pushups, then 30 second plank. Repeat for ten mins.	Squats and lunges for legs, push-ups for chest and arms, plank for core. (Modified as necessary to be right level for me)
Sunday morning swim	Sunday morning at local pool with a friend	30 minute swim – a mix of fast and slow lengths	Strengthen shoulder, back and leg muscles.

Endurance

What	When	How	Why
Family country walk	Saturday/ Sunday afternoon	1 hour walk in local countryside / park	Benefits of forest bathing. Time spent as a family. Can climb on fallen trees or play equipment for extra movement.
Sunday morning swim	Sunday morning at local pool with a friend	30 minute swim – a mix of fast and slow lengths	30 minutes of swimming is good endurance exercise for the heart and lungs.

How do I feel now?

Date	Energy level	Strength	Motivation
11 April	5/10	3/10	8/10
11 May	6/10	5/10	8/10

When you come up with your own plan, be realistic, but also be optimistic. Remember chapter eleven on self-identity? Who do you want to be and what are you working towards in terms of movement?

The plan looks like it has a lot of items on it, but as most are in the 'daily movement' section, they don't take up any time. These are habits you can build, and they don't cost any money at all.

Think about how you can make activities sociable and fun. The weekend swim and the country walk in the above example are with other people—but even if you are exercising alone, can you set up a group on a messenger app to keep you and your friends accountable and share tips and motivation?

When you have written your plan, set yourself a reminder to come back to it in one month's time. How is it going? Is it working for you? Do you feel any fitter? Compare the 'How do I feel now?' section to last month's.

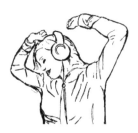

APPENDIX 2: WHAT NEW THING CAN I TRY?

If you fancy being a beginner at something, here's a list of all the different sports and activities that I can think of. Do any of these sound fun?

Aerobics

American football

Army basic training

Assault courses

Badminton

Ballet dancing

Ballroom dancing

Basketball

BMX

Bouldering

Boxing

Brazilian jiu jitzu

Breakdancing

Burlesque

Calisthenics

Capoeira

Caving

Circuit training

Circus skills

Cosplay / LARP

Cricket

Cross country skiing

Crossfit

Curling

Cycling

Diving

Dog agility

Energetic sex

Fencing

Football

Gardening

Geocaching

Golf

Gymnastics

High jump

HIIT

Hiking

Hockey

Horse riding

Hula hooping

Ice climbing

Ice skating

Javelin throwing

Jogging

Judo

Karate

Kayaking

Kickboxing

Kung fu

Lawn bowls

Less energetic sex

Lightsaber duelling

Long jump

Mixed martial arts

Mountain biking

Mountaineering

Netball

Nordic walking

Orienteering

Parkour

Pilates

Play on the kids' playground

Pokemon Go

Pole dancing

Prancercise (look it up)

Rock climbing

Roller skating

Roughhousing with your kids

Rounders

Rowing

Rugby

Sailing

Skateboarding

Skiing

Skipping rope

Snowboarding

Spinning

Sprinting

Squash

Stand up paddleboard

Street dance

Surfing

Swap your chair for a gym ball

Swimming in a pool

Swimming in open water

Sword fighting

Taekwondo

Tai Chi

Tap dancing

Tennis

Trampolining

Ultimate frisbee

Videogames you have to move for

Volleyball

Walking

Water aerobics

Water polo

Weightlifting

Yoga

Did I miss anything?

Further Reading (and Listening) and Endnotes

If I have inspired you to read any deeper into the ideas from other people in this book, the following are the best place to start:

Anything by **Katy Bowman**. My number one idol for moving and how to move. There are her books, *Move Your DNA, Movement Matters, Diastasis Recti...* plus there are literally thousands of hours of resources on her blog nutritiousmovement.com and she has a podcast: *Move Your DNA Podcast.*

Daniel Lieberman – *Exercised* (A big book about the evolution and science of exercise)

Gretchen Reynolds – *The First 20 Minutes* (A smaller book about the science of exercise)

Rangan Chatterjee – *Feel Better Live More* podcast: Dr Chatterjee interviews lots of different guests, including Daniel Lieberman and Tim Spector. There is an episode called *Why Walking is the Superpower You Never Knew You Had*, with Shane O'Mara, which will definitely inspire you to walk more), plus there are his books and resources on his website: drchatterjee.com

Tim Spector – for gut health and what to eat: *Spoon Fed* and *The Diet Myth*. Professor Spector is a co-founder of ZOE, a health science company that helps people improve their nutrition and ZOE has a podcast with episodes on exercise, the menopause, whether alcohol is good for you, and more: joinzoe.com/learn

The books mentioned are all available in audio format to listen to while on the move. The podcasts can be found wherever you like to listen to podcasts. For a real-life, physical book, may I suggest walking to your local library or independent bookshop to get hold of a copy, rather than ordering online? Libraries also have audiobooks available to borrow through the Borrowbox or Libby apps, so if you have a library card you can get free entertainment for while you move.

The easyfitnessforquitters.com website

On www.easyfitnessforquitters.com there are various resources to help you, including a Spotify playlist with hours of upbeat, fun music you can walk to, workout to, or just dance around the house to. See the *Resources* section for a template of the fitness plan for you to download and do with as you will. I have also included a huge list of different ways to move, and if you have any good tips and ideas, please add them to the comments!

1. Fatma Al-Maskari, MBChB, PhD, LRCP & SI, FFPH. United Nations Chronicle. www.un.org/en/chronicle/article/lifestyle-diseases-economic-burden-health-services.

2. NHS.uk. What is Type 2 Diabetes? www.nhs.uk/conditions/type-2-diabetes, 2020.

3. Lieberman, Daniel. Exercised. New York : Pantheon Books, a division of Penguin Random House, LLC, 2020.

4. Bullmore, Edward. The Inflamed Mind: A Radical New Approach to Depression. London : Short Books, 2018.

5. Lieberman, Daniel. Exercised. New York : Pantheon Books, a division of Penguin Random House, LLC, 2020.

6. Guedes, Luana Petruccio Cabral Moteiro, Cunha de Oliveira, Maria Liz and Carvalho, Gustavo de Azevedo. Deleterious effects of prolonged bed rest on the body systems of the elderly - a review. Universidade do Estado do Rio Janeiro : Revista Brasileira de Geriatria e Gerontologia, vol. 21, no. 4, 2018.

7. Harvard Health Publishing. Exercise is an all-natural treatment to fight depression. https://www.health.harvard.edu/mind-and-mood/exercise-is-an-all-natural-treatment-to-fight-depression, Harvard Medical School, 2021.

8. Reynolds, Gretchen. The First 20 Minutes: The surprising science of how we can exercise better, train smarter and live longer. London : Icon Books Ltd, 2013.

9. NHS.uk. Physical Activity Guidelines for Adults Aged 19 to 64. www.nhs.uk/live-well/exercise/exercise-guideli nes/physical-activity-guidelines-for-adults-aged -19-to-64, 2021.

10. Park Run is a free 5km (2km for juniors) community event that takes place every weekend in parks across the world. See www.parkrun.org.uk for more details.

11. Reynolds, Gretchen. The First 20 Minutes: The surprising science of how we can exercise better, train smarter and live longer. London : Icon Books Ltd, 2013.

12. Young, Damon. How to Think About Exercise. London : Macmillan, 2014.

13. Campaign to End Loneliness. The Facts on Loneliness. www.campaigntoendloneliness.org/the-facts-on -loneliness.

14. Lieberman, Daniel. Exercised. New York : Pantheon Books, a division of Penguin Random House, LLC, 2020.

15. NHS.uk. Walking for Health. www.nhs.uk/live-well/exercise/running-and-ae robic-exercises/walking-for-health, 2019.

16. Young, Damon. How to Think About Exercise. London : Macmillan, 2014.

17. Harvard Health Publishing. 5 surprising benefits of walking. www.health.harvard.edu/staying-healthy/5-surprising-benefits-of-walking, Harvard Medical School, 2021.

18. Lieberman, Daniel. Exercised. New York : Pantheon Books, a division of Penguin Random House, LLC, 2020.

19. Paluch, Amanda, Pettee Gabriel, Kelley and Fulton, Janet. Steps per Day and All-Cause Mortality in Middle-aged Adults in the Coronary Artery Risk Development in Young Adults Study. JAMA Network, 2021.

20. Paluch, Amanda, Pettee Gabriel, Kelley and Fulton, Janet. Steps per Day and All-Cause Mortality in Middle-aged Adults in the Coronary Artery Risk Development in Young Adults Study. JAMA Network, 2021.

21. Public Health England. Focus on brisk walking, not just 10,000 steps, say health experts. www.gov.uk/government/news/focus-on-brisk-walking-not-just-10000-steps-say-health-experts, 2018.

22. Bowman, Katy. The Best Walking Pace. www.nutritiousmovement.com/the-best-walking-pace.

23. House of Commons Library. Obesity Statistics. London : UK Parliament, 2022.

24. Wing, Rena R and Phelan, Suzanne. Long-term weight loss maintenance: The American Journal of Clinical Nutrition, Volume 82, Issue 1, 2005.

25. Wing, Rena R and Phelan, Suzanne. Long-term weight loss maintenance. The American Journal of Clinical Nutrition, Volume 82, Issue 1, 2005.

26. Newson, Dr. Louise. Mental health and emotional wellbeing in the perimenopause and menopause. Balance App Limited, 2022.

27. Bowman, Katy. My Pelvic Position in 2020. www.nutritiousmovement.com/my-pelvic-positi on-in-2020

28. Li, Q, et al. Effect of phytoncide from trees on human natural killer cell function. Tokyo, Japan : Int J Immunopathol Pharmacol, 2009.

29. Shanahan, D, Bush, R and Gaston, K. Health Benefits from Nature Experiences Depend on Dose, Sci Rep 6, 28551 h, 2016.

Acknowledgments

Thank you to the kind people who read various drafts of this book: Ross, Jenny A, Jenny B, Teresa, Michaela. Thank you to my parents for finding all the split infinitives. Who would have thought one book could contain so many? An especially big thank you to Mafe, who gave her time and writerly skill to go through the whole thing page by page with me. Kate Tilton in the US has also been hugely helpful, especially in showing me how to keep all the files organised, which is essential in self-publishing!

I owe thanks and gratitude beyond measure to Guy Windsor for his expertise in publishing and editing. I wouldn't have had the courage to go ahead and make the book a reality without his support. Guy, can I repay you in whisky and cigars?

And finally, thank you to my children for your help with getting my low-tech drawings sorted out and for insisting that I remove all the swear words. Top tip: if you need something done on a computer, ask a pre-teen.

About the Author

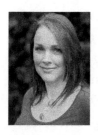 Katie Mackenzie trained as an emotional and performance coach as part of founding a social enterprise working with new parents. She has a knack for simplifying overwhelming or complicated concepts and a desire to help people feel better about themselves and less guilty about doing it wrong. Usually, there is no right or wrong.

She was inspired to write this book after chatting to a friend who bemoaned how unfit she felt and how unachievable getting into exercise seemed to be. Katie herself had been giving up on many, many, different exercise regimes over the years, as well as avidly learning about both physical and mental health. She felt it was time to bring it all together into a straightforward format to help others find motivation and enjoy movement.

Her favourite form of movement (this week) is long distance walking, especially with friends to chat to on the way and a stop for a picnic.

If you have enjoyed this book, please leave a review wherever you bought it from, or on www.easyfitnessforquitters.com. It really helps us authors spread the word about our books!

Thank you.

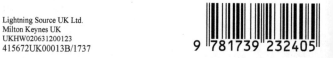